Exploring Transcultural Histories of Psychotherapies

This book draws together studies of the histories of psychotherapies throughout the world in a comparative setting, charting the intersections of these connected histories and transcultural networks of knowledge exchange and healing practices.

This volume's explorations of these transcultural histories help to illuminate the way in which these practices have shaped (and continue to shape) contemporary notions of psychological disorder, well-being, and identity itself. The contributors question the value-free status claimed by a wide array of contemporary psychotherapies, as well as the presuppositions of present-day 'evidence based' practice.

Suspended between several different fields, the advent of modern psychotherapies represents one of the distinctive features of twentieth-century Western societies, and one that has been rapidly spreading to other parts of the world. This volume will be of interest to those seeking to apply the conclusions of historical study to contemporary situations.

Chapters in this book were originally published in a special issue of *The European Journal of Psychotherapy & Counselling* or Taylor and Francis books.

Sonu Shamdasani is a Co-Director of the UCL Health Humanities Centre, London, UK. He works on the history of the psychological disciplines, with a particular focus on Jung's work and on the history of psychotherapies. He is the author and editor of numerous volumes, which have been translated into many languages.

Del Loewenthal is Emeritus Professor of Psychotherapy and Counselling at the University of Roehampton, London, UK. He is an existential-analytic psychotherapist, photographer, and chartered psychologist, with a particular interest in phenomenology. His books include *Existential Psychotherapy and Counselling after Postmodernism* (2017).

Exploring Transcultural Histories of Psychotherapies

Edited by
Sonu Shamdasani and Del Loewenthal

Routledge
Taylor & Francis Group

LONDON AND NEW YORK

First published 2020
by Routledge
2 Park Square, Milton Park, Abingdon, Oxon, OX14 4RN

and by Routledge
52 Vanderbilt Avenue, New York, NY 10017

Routledge is an imprint of the Taylor & Francis Group, an informa business

First issued in paperback 2021

British Library Cataloguing-in-Publication Data
A catalogue record for this book is available from the British Library

ISBN 13: 978-0-367-24686-0 (hbk)
ISBN 13: 978-1-03-208884-6 (pbk)

Typeset in Myriad Pro
by codeMantra

Publisher's Note
The publisher accepts responsibility for any inconsistencies that may
have arisen during the conversion of this book from journal articles to
book chapters, namely the inclusion of journal terminology.

Disclaimer
Every effort has been made to contact copyright holders for their
permission to reprint material in this book. The publishers would
be grateful to hear from any copyright holder who is not here
acknowledged and will undertake to rectify any errors or omissions in
future editions of this book.

Contents

Citation Information   vii
Notes on Contributors   ix

Introduction: Exploring Transcultural Histories of
Psychotherapies   1
Sonu Shamdasani and Del Loewenthal

1   Psychotherapy in Society: Historical reflections   8
    Sonu Shamdasani

2   Suggestion, persuasion and work: Psychotherapies in
    communist Europe   24
    Sarah Marks

3   Manualizing psychotherapy: Aaron T. Beck and the origins of
    Cognitive Therapy of Depression   39
    Rachael I. Rosner

4   Modernist Pills against Brazilian Alienism (1920–1945)   62
    Cristiana Facchinetti

5   Buddhism, Christianity, and psychotherapy: A three-way
    conversation in the mid-twentieth century   76
    Christopher Harding

6   Inferiority and bereavement: Implicit psychological
    commitments in the cultural history of Scottish psychotherapy   90
    Gavin Miller

7   Towards trans-cultural histories of psychotherapies   102
    Hans Pols

CONTENTS

8   Transcultural histories of psychotherapy   118
    Keir Martin

9   Therapy as cultural, politically influenced practice   134
    Del Loewenthal

    Index   149

Citation Information

The following chapters were originally published in *The European Journal of Psychotherapy & Counselling*, volume 20, issue 1 (March 2018). When citing this material, please use the original page numbering for each article, as follows:

Chapter 2
Suggestion, persuasion and work: Psychotherapies in communist Europe
Sarah Marks
The European Journal of Psychotherapy & Counselling, volume 20, issue 1 (March 2018) pp. 10–24

Chapter 3
Manualizing psychotherapy: Aaron T. Beck and the origins of Cognitive Therapy of Depression
Rachael I. Rosner
The European Journal of Psychotherapy & Counselling, volume 20, issue 1 (March 2018) pp. 25–47

Chapter 4
Modernist Pills against Brazilian Alienism (1920–1945)
Cristiana Facchinetti
The European Journal of Psychotherapy & Counselling, volume 20, issue 1 (March 2018) pp. 48–61

Chapter 5
Buddhism, Christianity, and psychotherapy: A three-way conversation in the mid-twentieth century
Christopher Harding
The European Journal of Psychotherapy & Counselling, volume 20, issue 1 (March 2018) pp. 62–75

Chapter 6

Inferiority and bereavement: Implicit psychological commitments in the cultural history of Scottish psychotherapy
Gavin Miller
The European Journal of Psychotherapy & Counselling, volume 20, issue 1 (March 2018) pp. 76–87

Chapter 7

Towards trans-cultural histories of psychotherapies
Hans Pols
The European Journal of Psychotherapy & Counselling, volume 20, issue 1 (March 2018) pp. 88–103

Chapter 8

Transcultural histories of psychotherapy
Keir Martin
The European Journal of Psychotherapy & Counselling, volume 20, issue 1 (March 2018) pp. 104–119

The following chapters were originally published in other Taylor and Francis books. When citing this material, please use the original information for each chapter, as follows:

Chapter 1

Psychotherapy in Society: Historical reflections
Sonu Shamdasani
Shamdasani, S. (2017). Chapter 20, 'Psychotherapy in Society: Historical reflections', pp. 363–378 in Eghigian, G. (ed.) The Routledge History of Madness and Mental Health. Oxon: Routledge.

Chapter 9

Therapy as cultural, politically influenced practice
Del Loewenthal
Loewenthal, D. (2016). Chapter 1, 'Therapy as cultural, politically influenced practice', in Lees, J. (ed.) The future of psychological therapy: Managed care, practitioner research and clinical innovation. Oxon: Routledge. [This is a revised version.]

For any permission-related enquiries please visit:
http://www.tandfonline.com/page/help/permissions

Contributors

Cristiana Facchinetti is a Researcher in the Research Department and a Professor of the Postgraduate Program in History of Science and Health at the Casa de Oswaldo Cruz, Brazil. Her research and teaching interests include the history of global mental health; the history of psychiatry, disease, and poverty in Brazilian social thought; and the history of Psychoanalysis and its impact on Brazilian culture.

Christopher Harding is a Senior Lecturer in Asian History at the University of Edinburgh, UK. He works on the cultural history of modern India and Japan, with a particular interest in religion, spirituality, and mental health.

Del Loewenthal is Emeritus Professor of Psychotherapy and Counselling at the University of Roehampton, London, UK. He is an existential-analytic psychotherapist, photographer, and chartered psychologist, with a particular interest in phenomenology.

Sarah Marks is a Lecturer in Modern History and a UKRI Future Leaders Fellow at Birkbeck, University of London, UK. Her research focuses on the history of the psy-disciplines during the cold war.

Keir Martin is an Associate Professor of Social Anthropology at the University of Oslo, Norway, and is a member of the British Association for Counselling and Psychotherapy. His research interests include psychotherapy and the changing nature of corporate governance.

Gavin Miller is a Senior Lecturer in Medical Humanities at the University of Glasgow, UK. His research interests include the critical history of psychotherapy, and the connections between science fiction and psychological discourse.

Hans Pols is a Professor and the Head of the School of History and Philosophy of Science at the University of Sydney, Australia. His research focuses on global mental health, and the history of psychology, psychiatry, and psychotherapy.

Rachael I. Rosner is an Independent Scholar in Boston, USA. Her general historical interest is in twentieth-century American psychotherapy, with particular focus on Aaron T Beck's cognitive therapy and on post-war ego psychology.

Sonu Shamdasani is a Co-Director of the UCL Health Humanities Centre, London, UK. He works on the history of the psychological disciplines, with a particular focus on Jung's work and on the history of psychotherapies.

Exploring Transcultural Histories of Psychotherapies

Sonu Shamdasani and Del Loewenthal

We will build a groundbreaking psychological therapy service in England. Backed by new investment rising to £170 million by 2010–11, the service will be capable of treating 900,000 additional patients suffering from depression and anxiety over the next three years. Around half are likely to be completely cured, with many fewer people with mental health problems having to depend on sick pay and benefits. Gordon Brown, 10 October 2007.[1]

The so-called Improving Access to Psychological Therapies (IAPT) which Gordon Brown announced had been the result of an initiative by Richard Layard, an economist and Labour peer, and David Clark, a Cognitive Behavioural Therapist.[2] The argument that Clark and Layard put forward was recently restated in their book, *Thrive: The Power of Evidence-Based Psychological Therapies*. They begin by marshalling an array of statistics, noting that in 2008, the World Health Organisation estimated that in wealthy countries, "mental illness accounts for nearly 40% of all illness. By contrast, stroke, cancer, heart disease, lung disease and diabetes account for under 20%."[3] More than half of this is comprised of depression and anxiety. As to the proportion of the population thus afflicted, they cite statistics which claim that 27% of the population in the EU suffer in some way from mental illness.[4] They further noted that in the UK the economic cost of mental illness amounted to 7% of national income, but we spend 1% of national income to treat it. Only 13% of the health budget spent on mental health, which constituted a "system-level discrimination."[5] The solution to this lay ready to hand in the form of Cognitive Behaviour Therapy (CBT) which they claimed has brought "psychological therapy to a point where it can claim scientifically to be able to transform lives."[6] The persuasiveness of their argument was based on the claim that a short course of CBT would easily pay for itself through reducing economic costs borne by the state due to mental disorders.

The history of psychotherapy that Clark and Layard provide is a simple tale with a happy ending: Chapter 1, "In the beginning was Freud. He was the founder of talking therapies – and in particular of listening therapies. He, more than anyone, taught therapists how to listen ... However psychoanalysis has not been shown to be effective."[7] Chapter 2: Aaron Beck rides to the rescue with the formulation of CBT, which is the first form of psychotherapy to demonstrate its effectiveness via the evidence-based gold standard of randomised clinical trials. By 2011, IAPT had been rolled out to treat 400,000 people and a further £400 million was pledged, with the aim to treat a further 2.6 million by 2015. The department of health claimed that the £400 million expenditure would result in savings of £700 million to the public sector in healthcare, tax, and welfare gains.[8] CBT was thus one of the coalition's more unusual means of trying to reduce the deficit. As has readily been apparent, such massive state investment in and legitimation of one particular form of psychotherapy above others has had massive implications for the ecosystem of the wider psychotherapeutic field, imbricating its micropolitics with the macropolitics of government.

In the field of mental health, we are familiar with the use of statistics for rhetorical purposes, without indicating precisely how they are derived, and the often questionable assumptions behind them. However, the scale of these figures coupled with the mass-rollout of the antidote in the form of psychotherapies renders timely historical inquiry into psychotherapies, and the study of how they have come to occupy the positions that they hold within contemporary societies. In short, to replace Clark and Layard's legitimating myth of origins with historical inquiry and interrogation.[9]

First, one may ask, as further explored in Chapter 1, what is psychotherapy? The term has been applied to almost any form of conversation between two individuals with an aim to enabling a therapeutic change in one of them. The definitional problem poses particular challenges for histories of psychotherapies: not only is one faced with the difficulty of selecting one's object of study, this choice may play an active role in determining the very identity of the object itself, akin to a historical indeterminacy principle: witness, for example, the active role of historiography in constituting psychoanalysis.[10] Furthermore, psychotherapeutic idioms have come to inhabit the vernacular and seep into other spheres. Consequently, histories of psychotherapies must by necessity overflow discrete disciplinary trajectories, and broach broader socio-cultural transformations that these practices have given rise to.

Suspended between science, medicine, religion, art, and philosophy, the advent of modern psychotherapies represents one of the distinctive features of twentieth-century Western societies, and they are increasing being exported to the rest of the world. However, their historical study glaringly lags behind their societal impact and the role they play in contemporary mental health policies in a number of countries. In recent years, a small but significant body of work has arisen studying histories of psychotherapies in discrete local contexts throughout the world, which is expanding and reframing our knowledge of them. However, little has been done to draw this work together within a comparative setting, and to chart the intersection of these connected histories and transcultural networks of exchange of knowledge and healing practices. There are signs that this situation is changing.[11]

But how should this study be undertaken? Some of the complexities can be seen through considering the current situation in China. In 2012, China passed its first mental health act, which placed in statute the task of promoting psychological well-being and preventing mental disorders. The act provided state recognition of psychotherapy and psychological counselling, and required medical facilities to provide psychotherapeutic services. The act was clear that psychotherapy was to be regarded as a medical speciality, but was silent on providing further details as to what psychotherapy is, leaving the task of the "technical regulations for the provision of psychotherapy [to] the administrative departments for health under the State Council."[12] Anthropologists have spoken of a 'psychotherapy fever' currently spreading across China.[13] In recent decades, it has been a burgeoning export market for European and American styles of psychotherapy, subject to complex patterns of interpretation and adaptation. This in turn has posed numerous questions concerning the relation of Western psychotherapy to Chinese thought. Some have argued that "indigenous forms of psychotherapy have existed in China for centuries," retrospectively recategorising Chinese medical traditions.[14] Such questions are not only historical: witness the mirror developments of mindfulness-based therapies in the West and of Daoist Cognitive Psychotherapy in China.

In such contexts, the question pressingly rises, what exactly is being imported? If one looks to the proponents of the import drive, one can get some clear answers: psychotherapy, it is maintained, represents universally applicable methods of treatment based in turns on universal and scientifically validated models of the mind. As we are familiar 'the West' has been taken as a synonym for 'the universal.' From this angle, the task of a global history of psychotherapy would simply be one of mapping its origins and subsequent geographical spread. However, such a project would simply represent uncritically subscribing to the assumptions that underlie contemporary Western psychotherapies. By contrast, in developing a transcultural perspective on the history of psychotherapy, rather than a global history, what is required is a provincialising approach, to borrow a term from Dipesh Chakrabarty. As he put it: "to provincialize Europe is precisely to find out how and in what sense European ideas that were universal were also at one and the same time drawn from very particular intellectual traditions that could not claim any universal validity."[15] Only by excavating the cultural and temporal embeddedness of Western psychotherapy is one in a position to understand what is subsequently being transferred and adapted to radically different cultural contexts. In the practice of translation, one commonly regards the integrity and identity of the source text as sacrosanct. Paradoxically, in case of cultural transmission, the very act of translation can confer a stable identity to an object which it lacks in its original cultural context. Here, one cannot presuppose the existence of a stable source 'text' to be unproblematically transferred to a target 'language,' particularly as what is being transferred are not only theories but practices embedded in particular cultural nexuses, involving tacit assumptions, implicit 'know how,' cultural cues, and ritualised forms of hieratic transmission of what Michael Balint memorably referred to as the 'apostolic function.'[16] Consequently, what replication can mean in such situations is rendered quite muddy.[17] In place of a centre to periphery model, what is required is the study of, as Kapil Raj puts it, reciprocal processes of circulation and negotiation.[18] Thus, comparative provincialising provides productive opportunities for reciprocal reworkings of monadic histories. Consequently, transcultural histories of psychotherapies would at the same time chart how psychotherapeutic practices have come to transform cultures.

The chapters that follow trace some of these routes, highlighting nodal points and intersections, while remaining mindful of the manner in which histories have been used to construct the very identity of the field. What emerges is no single narrative, but rather a series of connections and contrasts, conjunctions and disjunctions, which jointly fracture monolithic narratives of the rise of psychotherapies.

Turning now to the plan of this book. Following our above introduction, this volume commences by addressing methodological issues in carrying out comparative histories on these stories amongst stories. Chapter 1 'Psychotherapy in Society: Historical reflections' is by Shamdasani. He considers 'what is psychotherapy?' arguing that any historical enquiry into this subject must begin by posing this question.

The following five chapters were originally published in *The European Journal of Psychotherapy and Counselling* (issue 20.01, March 2018). These chapters arose from a conference at the UCL Health Humanities Centre in 2016, "Towards Transcultural Histories of Psychotherapies," made possible by the support of the UCL Global Engagement Office. (The conference marked the inception of the Transcultural Histories of Psychotherapy Project, which seeks to promote research in this field through convening workshops and conferences, and fostering exchanges and collaborations. For more information see www.historiesofpsychotherapy.net.)

Chapter 2, the first of these five chapters, is 'Suggestion Persuasion and Work: Psychotherapies in communist Europe' by Sarah Marks. She provides a historical account of the various developments in the field of psychotherapy in Communist Europe. She offers a historical parallel between the development of suggestion and persuasion psychotherapy models in the East and West, arguing that psychotherapy, in various modalities and at different levels of visibility, has had a larger presence and influence in communist Europe than is typically given credit.

In Chapter 3, 'Manualizing psychotherapy: Aaron T. Beck and the origins of Cognitive Therapy of Depression,' Rachael Rosner presents some insights into Aaron Beck's development of treatment manuals for cognitive therapy. She draws upon rich material from interviews with leading figures in the field. She also refers to the contemporary debate about the manualisation of psychotherapy.

Cristiana Facchinetti in Chapter 4, 'Modernist Pills against Brazilian Alienism,' provides a contribution to the study and circulation of transnational knowledge and practices. She covers a wide range of ideas relating to Brazilian cultural as well as its intellectual and political history. She argues that psychoanalysis was appropriated by Brazilian Avant-Garde intellectuals, as an attempt to counter cultural colonialism within Brazil.

Chapter 5 entitled 'Buddhism, Christianity, and Psychotherapy: A Three-Way Conversation in the Mid-Twentieth Century' by Christopher Harding adds to the developments of contemporary psychotherapy. He investigates the processes, associations, and potential pitfalls that arise in the dialogue between psychotherapy and religion, with a focus on Buddhism. Psychotherapy is approached critically as part of the 'psy-complex' – the set of contemporary institutional practices that concerns the making and regulation of modern Western personhood. Some of its associations with one trend, drawing upon the work of Kosawa Keisaku, of Japanese Buddhism and Christianity are discussed.

Chapter 6, 'Inferiority and bereavement: Implicit psychological commitments in the cultural history of Scottish psychotherapy,' is by Gavin Miller. He considers methodological issues in his historiographic research on psychoanalytic psychotherapy in Scotland. Taking Scotland as a case study, the author argues that psychotherapy in Scotland adapted to a culture context which chose to integrate psychotherapy together with a critique of religion by the human sciences, which in turn impelled a belief in the scientifically rational.

What then follows are two Chapters 7 and 8, commissioned through *The European Journal of Psychotherapy & Counselling*, which are responses to Chapters 2–6. The first, Chapter 7, is from Hans Pols. In his response towards 'Transcultural Histories of Psychotherapy,' he argues that tracing the transnational and transcultural dissemination of psychotherapy enables historians 'to chart their inherent variability, test limits, and analyse its broader social and political uses.'

The second respondent is Keir Martin, who in Chapter 8 also questions the assumption of psychotherapy's origins as a Western practice. He argues that not only will Bangalore and Shanghai rival Hampstead and Manhattan as centres influencing therapeutic practice and theory, but that we will in future need to pay far more attention to the 'culture concept' in different contexts.

The final chapter, Chapter 9, is 'Therapy as Cultural, Politically Influenced Practice' by Del Loewenthal. He shows how such decisions from the UK's National Institute of Clinical Excellence (NICE) on the recommended provision for those suffering from depression is not a purely scientific process.

Our particular thanks to all these contributors to this book and to Akihito Suzuki, who open up productive new perspectives in this societally significant, but under-researched field. As well as new lines of historical research and transcultural comparison across and between different contexts, it is hoped through more cultural considerations, as described in this book, new possibilities will emerge in the present. For example, Western psychotherapeutic practitioners and researchers may have a better means to grasp the local situatedness and lack of universality of their theoretical models, and question their psychotherapies' ethnocentrism (let alone their dubious attempts at scientific legitimacy) as may those in other countries that are now importing such Western ideas to their very different contexts.

Notes

1. Hansard, 10 October 2007, available at www.parliament.uk.
2. Layard's father incidentally was John Layard, a noted anthropologist and Jungian analyst, as well as being a serial patient. He underwent therapy with around 20 therapists in the course of his life, including Homer Lane, H. G. Baynes, Siegfried Bernfeld, Wilhelm Stekel, Fritz Wittels, Erna Rosenbaum, Gerhard Adler, C. G. Jung and R. D. Laing. See Jeremy McClanchy, "Unconventional character and disciplinary convention: John Layard, Jungian and anthropologist," in George Stocking ed., *Malinowski, Rivers, Benedict and Others: Essays on Culture and Personality*, (Madison, University of Wisconsin Press, 1988), pp. 50–71.
3. David Clark and Richard Layard, *Thrive: The Power of Evidence-Based Psychological Therapies*, (London, Penguin, 2014), p. 5.
4. *Ibid.*, p. 39.
5. *Ibid.*, pp. 87–88.
6. *Ibid.*, p. 10. On the history of CBT in Britain, see Sarah Marks, "Cognitive behaviour therapies in Britain: the historical context and present situation," in Ed. Windy Dryden, Cognitive Behaviour Therapies (London, Sage, 2012), pp. 1–25.
7. *Ibid.*, p. 131.
8. *IAPT Three Year Report: The First Million Patients*, Department of Health, 2012, available at: www.dh.gsi.gov.uk.
9. On the new historiography of psychotherapy, see Sarah Marks, "Psychotherapy in historical perspective," *History of the Human Sciences* 2017, 30(2), pp. 3–16.
10. See Mikkel Borch-Jacobsen and Sonu Shamdasani, *The Freud Files: An Inquiry into the History of Psychoanalysis*, (Cambridge, Cambridge University Press, 2012).
11. In 2013, the Centre for the History of the Psychological Disciplines at UCL (now the Health Humanities Centre) held a conference "From Moral Treatment to Psychological Therapies: Psychotherapeutics from the York Retreat to the Present Day" organised by Sarah Marks. Some of the chapters from this have now appeared in a special issue of *History of the Human Sciences* on "Psychotherapy in Historical Perspective" (30, 2, 2017), guest editor, Sarah Marks. A complementary special issue of *History of Psychology* (21, 3, 2018) on psychotherapy in the Americas was edited by Rachael Rosner. In 2017, Gavin Miller organised a conference at the University of Glasgow on "Other Psychotherapies: Psychotherapies across Time, Space and Cultures." A special issue of *Transcultural Psychiatry*, guest editor Gavin Miller, is forthcoming.
12. H.H. Chen, M.R. Phillips, H. Cheng, Q.Q. Chen, X.D. Chen, D. Fralick, Y.E. Zhang, M. Liu, J. Huang, and M. Bueber, "Mental Health Law of the People's Republic of China (English translation with annotations)" *Shanghai Archives of Psychiatry*, 24(6), 2012, pp. 305–321.
13. "It's good to talk: China opens up to psychotherapy," *The Guardian*, 3 September, 2014.
14. John K. Miller and Xiaoyi Fang, "Marriage and Family Therapy in the People's Republic of China: Current Issues and Challenges," *Journal of Family Psychotherapy*, 23, pp. 173–183.

15. Dipesh Chakrabarty, *Provincializing Europe: Postcolonial Thought and Historical Difference*, (Princeton, Princeton University Press, 2007), p. xiii.
16. Michael Balint, *The Doctor, His Patient and the Illness*, (London, Pitman Medical Publishing, 1957); Shaul Bar-Heim, "'The apostolic function': Michael Balint and the postwar GP," UCL/British Psychological Society History of the Psychological Disciplines Seminar, UCL Health Humanities Centre, 15 February 2016.
17. On the problematic of replication in science studies, see Harry Collins, *Changing Order: Replication and Induction in Scientific Practice*, (London, Sage, 1985).
18. Kapil Raj, *Relocating Modern Science: Circulation and the Construction of Knowledge in South Asia and Europe 1650–1900*, (London, Palgrave Macmillan, 2007).

PSYCHOTHERAPY IN SOCIETY
Historical reflections

Sonu Shamdasani

What is psychotherapy? Any historical inquiry into the subject must begin by posing this question. One of the earliest definitions from 1892 by the Dutch psychiatrist Frederick van Eeden (1869–1932), ran as follows: 'I call psychotherapy all curative methods which use psychic agents to combat illness through the intervention of psychic functions.'[1] This was a wide, all-embracing definition, simply setting aside the body. Half a century later, Karl Jaspers (1883–1969) proposed the following: 'Psychotherapy is the name given to all those methods of treatment that affect both psyche and body by measures which proceed via the psyche. The co-operation of the patient is always required.'[2] Little had changed. In 1973, Thomas Szasz (1920–2012) attempted to gather together the plethora of definitions into one:

> We have come to accept as psychotherapy all conceivable situations in which the soul, spirit, mind, or personality of an individual who claims to be a healer is employed to bring about some sort of change called 'therapeutic' in the soul, spirit, mind or personality of another individual, called the 'patient'.[3]

Given the breadth and vagueness of what is covered by these definitions, it is fruitful to begin with consideration of the term itself.

In 1853, a surgeon to the royal infirmary for diseases of children in London and former president of the medical society, Walter Cooper Dendy (1794–1871), published a book entitled *Psyche: A Discourse on the Birth and Pilgrimage of Thought*, in which he described 'psychotherapeia' as the 'antidote of thought'.[4] For Dendy, psychotherapeia represented the use of the remedial influence of the mind: 'We know how instantaneously a thought will stimulate the salivary, the spermatic and other glands.'[5] As mental states induced disorder, prevention and cure could be brought about by inducing a contrary state of mind. Dendy was in effect referring to the long-standing medicine of the imagination. The following year, an anonymous reviewer of Forbes Winslow's *Lectures on Insanity* in the *Asylum Journal* referred to the moral and medical treatment of insanity as the 'the twin brothers of the psychotherapeutic art, the Castor and Pollux of mental medicine'.[6] The reference here was clearly to moral treatment.

The term was picked up two decades later by Daniel Hack Tuke (1827–1895) in 1872. A psychiatrist and the great-grandson of William Tuke, the founder of the York Retreat, he used the term 'psycho-therapeutics' in his *Illustrations of the Influence of the Mind Upon the Body in Health and Disease Designed to Elucidate the Action of the Imagination*.[7] He claimed that physicians had long known the healing power of the imagination, but that now it could be made rational. This would serve to distinguish them from quacks – the latter being individuals who healed without knowing how they did so. The spectre of quackery has haunted psychotherapy, and most schools have commenced by arguing why they (as opposed to their rivals) should not be regarded as quacks. The penultimate chapter of Tuke's book was titled 'Psycho-Therapeutics – Practical Applications of the Influence of the Mind on the Body to Medical Practice'. Whilst discussing animal magnetism, he argued that the 1784 French Commission on animal magnetism were correct in attributing the phenomena that they observed to the effect of the imagination and imitation, and that this could form the basis of a new science, 'that of the Moral over the Physical'.[8] For Tuke, mesmerism thus displayed how 'certain purely psychical agencies produce certain physical results'.[9] Whilst boldly proclaiming the new science of psycho-therapeutics, Tuke appears not to have made further use of the term.

It might well have ended there, had it not caught the attention of Hippolyte Bernheim (1840–1919). A professor of medicine at Nancy, he had become interested in the work of Auguste Ambroise Liébault (1823–1904), a country doctor who practised hypnosis. According to Bernheim, it was Liébault who established 'the doctrine of therapeutic suggestion'.[10] Bernheim claimed that suggestion was as 'old as the world'.[11] What was new was its systematic application to therapeutics. For Bernheim, the use of suggestion not only featured prominently in his practice, it formed the theoretical key to understanding hypnosis and a general psychology of the mind. Hypnosis was understood as a state of heightened suggestibility, akin to sleep. He defined suggestion widely, as the act by which an idea is accepted in the brain. For Bernheim and the Nancy school, suggestive therapeutics consisted in the deliberate manipulation of credence, belief, and expectation under the rubric of suggestion and autosuggestion in the treatment of a wide range of psychological and physical conditions. In addition to functional neuroses, Bernheim claimed that it was effective in cases of paralyses, contractures, insomnia, muscular pain, hemiplegia, paraplegia, rheumatism, anaesthesia, gastric disorders, neuralgia, and sciatica. The common factor active in religious healing as well as in many therapeutic practices, was held to be suggestion.[12] Thus 'suggestion' was presented as a modern rational scientific concept which both explained and unmasked prior and contemporary medical therapies and forms of religious healing. Individuals flocked to Nancy to visit Bernheim and Liébault and watch them at work and gain instruction in hypnosis. Nancy became a 'medical Mecca'.[13] A hypnotic movement spread rapidly through Europe. A controversy raged between the Nancy school and the Salpêtrière school, under the neurologist Jean-Martin Charcot (1825–1893). For Charcot and his followers, hypnosis was only found in cases of hysteria. What Charcot described as 'grand hypnotisme' followed three stages, each of which had distinct physiological characteristics: catalepsy, lethargy, and somnambulism. At the Salpêtrière, Charcot used hypnosis to study the underlying architecture of hysteria; because he claimed it was a pathological state, he was not interested in its therapeutic applications.[14]

Addressing the conflict that raged between the hypnotic schools, the Belgian philosopher and hypnotist Joseph Delboeuf (1831–1896) stated that in addition to the well-known influence of the hypnotiser on the hypnotised, the influence in the reciprocal direction was critical.[15] The subjects, generally the first or paradigm case, trained the experimenter and influenced his methods without his realising it.

This set up a template, as the experimenter reported his results to his disciples who 'replicated' them. It was this circuit of reciprocal influence which gave rise to the hypnotic schools, each monopolising special phenomena. Delboeuf claimed that it was impossible for the experimenter to situate himself outside of the field of effects of the suggestive influence they were attempting to objectively study. His critique suggested that the respective hypnotic schools had become veritable influencing machines for the generation of evidence. The fact that different traits could be paraded forth as constituting the essence of hypnosis and appear to gain confirmation from other practitioners indicated that the mode of institutionalisation was itself subject to the effects of hypnosis and suggestion, which could not be neutralised. The conflicts between the various schools were insolvable, for each of them could point to evidence that supported their particular theories.

In 1886, in the second expanded edition of his book, Bernheim took up the term from Tuke, whose book had just appeared in French.[16] Citing Tuke, Bernheim referred to the 'psycho-therapeutic action' of suggestion and the 'hypnotic psycho-therapeutic'.[17] As Tuke's term had been adopted as a synonym, there was no need for a separate definition of psycho-therapeutics. It was through the hypnotic movement that the term psychotherapy became rapidly disseminated in an open source manner and was widely adopted. Psychotherapy rode on the back of the burgeoning hypnotic movement; consequently there was no need for a separate definition of it. The genie quickly escaped from the bottle, and through the Nancy school discussion of suggestion rapidly entered popular culture, as questions concerning mental influence, the limits of free will, the hidden powers of the mind, the nature of the social bond, the basis of political organisation and religious authority. The theory of suggestion became the lynchpin of a new ontology.

This in turn set up a feedback loop that affected the very practice itself. As Delboeuf pointed out, it had become rare to encounter a naive subject, who has never heard discussion of magnetism or hypnotism. Subjects were already being schooled by society at large. Subjects had preconceived ideas, from conversations or lectures or public demonstrations, which influenced their conduct and set up expectations that in turn structured the therapeutic encounter – ruling out of question the possibility of a naive empiricism – and one which still forms the basis of outcome studies in psychotherapy today. Delboeuf drew the radical conclusion that hypnosis did not exist, or, in other words, that 'the power of hypnotism consists above all in the very word of hypnotism, because [the subject] does not understand it well'.[18] The term itself had a suggestive effect.

Critically, as hypnosis increasingly fell into disrepute, the term psychotherapy presented itself as a ready alternative for an eclectic mix of practices. The decline of hypnosis was accompanied by a revival of moral therapy. A prominent advocate of this was Paul Dubois (1884–1918), a Swiss physician and professor of neuropathology in Bern. In 1904, he published the extremely popular *Psychoneuroses and Their Moral Treatment.* Dubois launched a critique of suggestion, claiming that it only increased the state of servitude of patients. Psychoneurotics needed to be immunised from suggestion, so that they would accept 'nothing but the councils of reason'.[19] Patients needed to regain their self-mastery. In place of suggestion, he spoke of moral persuasion. Critically, Dubois took up the term psychotherapy, seeking to dissociate it from suggestive therapeutics.[20] For him, it was Pinel who 'first introduced psychotherapy in the treatment of mental diseases'.[21] Liébault and Bernheim, and the whole magnetic and hypnotic traditions, were displaced. The implications were clear: psychotherapy was simply the modern form of moral treatment.[22]

Whilst Bernheim had stressed the application of suggestion – and hence psycho-therapy – to physical and what would today be classed as psychosomatic disorders, the purview of psychotherapy became increasingly restricted to the 'psychoneuroses'. Dubois argued that he commenced by eliminating the neuroses with a probable somatic origin, restricting himself to 'neurasthenia, hysteria, hystero-neurasthenia, the light forms of hypochondria and melancholy [and . . .] certain more serious states of disequilibrium, such as vesania'.[23] The conditions noted by Dubois do not feature in contemporary diagnostic manuals. Part of the longevity of psychotherapy as a profession has resided in its effectiveness in ever formulating and catering for new disorders.[24]

In 1904, Jean Camus and Philippe Pagniez presented a history of psychotherapy. They differentiated between the conscious manifestations of psychotherapy and its unconscious use. They argued that both modalities went back to antiquity and arranged their history thematically under four headings: psychotherapy by remedies, by which they meant 'suggestion by medicinal therapeutics'; psychotherapy by 'the marvellous' (understood as the intervention of supernatural beings); psychotherapy by hypnotism and suggestion; and psychotherapy by persuasion. If psychotherapy was nothing new, the value of the present was one of 'determining its mechanism of action, of making its usage precise and of grouping together all the scattered rules and indications'.[25]

By the beginning of the twentieth century, the word 'psychotherapy' had become firmly established, but it was not the exclusive preserve of any one figure or school. It was variously adopted to refer to a variety of procedures, ranging from mesmerism, hypnosis, suggestive therapy, moral therapy, Mind-Cure, mental healing, strengthening of the will, reeducation, the cathartic method, rational per-suasion, to general medical practice or the 'art' of medicine. Histories had started to be written and contested. A heterogeneous cluster of therapeutic practices to be grouped together under the term, identified as a modern, rational, scientific discipline. This pre-staged its development in the twentieth century and the vast range of denotation that it acquired. The term was adopted by an array of diver-gent practices and disciplines, a development facilitated by the fact that it never was one thing.

Thus psychotherapy has no one origin, no one clear genealogy. One can begin a history of psychotherapy almost wherever one likes – which is reflected in the liter-ature on the topic. We find no consensus regarding which millennia to commence with, let alone century. We are confronted then with a series of 'connected histories', to adopt Sanjay Subrahmanyan's term, which come together, intersect, and branch apart.[26] 'Psychotherapy' is a set of historically situated practices, which both embody and produce specific cultural values. Rather than presupposing an essence at the level of the referent, one needs to follow the circulation, exchange, and shifting modalities of a network of related practices in different domains. What follows then is simply an attempt to trace some of these routes, highlighting certain nodal points and intersec-tions, while remaining mindful of the manner in which histories have been used to construct the very identity of the field.

In the twentieth century, psychotherapy was an ontology-making practice.[27] The therapeutic encounter became a site where individuals not only were cured, or not, as the case might be; but also learnt to articulate their suffering in new idioms, reconceive their lives according to particular narrative templates, and take on conceptions concerning the nature of the mind and reality. The consequence of this has been the generation of a plethora of optional ontologies. These have come to encompass world views, codes of conduct, and, at times, full-blown soteriologies or systems of salvation. A history of psychotherapies then, informs us not only about the history of discrete therapeutic practices, but also how psychotherapies have generated new conceptions of the mind, conduct, and behaviour that were, and continue to be, taken up by the public at large.

For Bernheim, the practice of psychotherapy was an outpatient medical procedure that used existing medical nosologies. From the 1890s onwards, there was a rapid expansion of the notion of functional nervous disorders, or the neuroses. From here on, psychotherapy was to minister to its own set of proprietary ailments; furthermore, each school increasingly came to have its own set. The central figure in this regard was Pierre Janet. Janet (1857–1947) initially trained in philosophy. From 1883 to 1889, he taught at Le Havre and commenced studying hypnosis and suggestion. Janet's investigations resulted in a series of landmark articles, culminating in 1889 in *Psychological Automatism*.[28] He presented a position between that of the Nancy and Salpêtrière schools. He articulated his model of the dissociation of consciousness and the role of the subconscious. Whilst these terms were already in use, they became firmly associated with Janet. For Janet, hypnosis offered an experimental means to study the personality. It demonstrated the existence of separate memory chains, or 'automatisms', which could go as far as to form alternate or double personalities. For Janet, the dissociation of consciousness formed an explanation of suggestion, hypnotic and post-hypnotic states, as well as hysteria. Janet referred to the subconscious as opposed to the unconscious as the acts in question, whilst not 'conscious' to the primary consciousness, were 'conscious' to the secondary consciousness.

Continuing his research under Charcot at the Salpêtrière hospital in Paris, he completed his medical studies in 1893 with a dissertation, *The Mental States of Hysterics*.[29] That year, Charcot opened a psychological laboratory at the Salpêtrière, which he entrusted to Janet. Developing Charcot's research, Janet viewed hysteria as a psychogenic disorder, characterised by a narrowing of the field of personal consciousness and a tendency to the dissociation of sensations and memories. These dissociated memories and sensations continued to exist in the subconscious and have effects. He laid particular emphasis on the pathogenic effect of traumatic events in lives of patients and held that they could be led to recollect such events under hypnosis, automatic writing, and crystal gazing.

During this period, Janet paid attention to dreams and subconscious reveries. The therapeutic significance of the former was that they often revealed the pathogenic event, and brought to light subconscious fixed ideas that could subsequently be liquidated. With the sick, subconscious reveries became involuntary, and Janet characterised hysterics as individuals who, not content to dream at night, dreamt all day long. Neurotics had the need to be directed, and this role had to be assumed by the physician, in order for the patient to regain their self-mastery. Janet called his method 'psychological analysis'. In Vienna, Breuer and Freud drew upon Janet's work, and a priority dispute later broke out between them. Subsequent historical research has tended to support Janet's claims. In 1902, he succeeded Théodule Ribot in his post at the Collège de France. Though prominent in his lifetime, Janet never formed a school or movement and did not cultivate disciples. Janet's conception of the dissociation of consciousness was widely taken up. In many respects, the pathological psychology which he developed had its greatest impact on the burgeoning field of psychotherapy. Through the effects of the Freudian legend, much that should have been attributed to his work was instead ascribed to psychoanalysis.

In 1903, Janet reflected on the social historical significance of psychotherapy. He observed that when patients found a friend or someone whom they could obey, their problems ceased. He argued that priests had formerly fulfilled this function, and doctors could now do the same. Priests had done this in a haphazard manner, and no longer had the authority that they once had: 'It is a characteristic of our time that this work of moral direction has sometimes returned to the doctor, who is now often charged with this role of moral direction when the patient does not find enough support around him.'[30] This notion of psychotherapy as fulfilling a function previously served by the Church became increasingly significant in the decades that followed, particularly in the work of Jung, alongside attempts to combine psychotherapy with pastoral care.[31]

In 1919, Janet published his *Psychological Medications*, which presented a seminally important account of the history of psychotherapy combined with a full articulation of his new system, recasting his earlier studies in the light of the latter.[32] It presented an elaborate new model of psychotherapy, underpinned by psychological energetics. It was never taken up in the manner in which his early studies of dissociation had and continue to be taken up. However, his account of the relations of magnetic tradition to the hypnotic tradition provided one of the main templates for how it has been subsequently viewed.[33] In a similar manner to Bernheim, he held to the negative model of the goal of psychotherapy, as the removal of pathology. For him, it constituted the totality of physical and mental procedures applied to mental and bodily disorders through consideration of psychological phenemona. It thus represented the application of psychological science to the treatment of disease.[34]

For decades, we have laboured under the spell of the Freud legend, which has led to the wholesale mystification of the history of psychotherapy.[35] Freud started as a neurologist in private practice, and, as was common, utilised electrotherapy and the Weir Mitchell rest cure. In 1885, he went to study with Charcot in Paris and became interested in hysteria. In 1893, Freud, published, together with his senior colleague and mentor, Josef Breuer, 'On the Psychical Mechanism of Hysteria: Preliminary Communication'.[36] At this time, a number of figures were interested in issues related to catharsis in psychotherapy. Breuer and Freud argued that the symptoms of hysteria were due to a precipitating trauma. They represented symbolic connections, for example, vomiting after experiencing feeling of mental disgust. In effect, they were expanding and generalising Charcot's concept of traumatic hysteria and notion of 'passionate attitudes'. They argued that in hysteria, the psychical trauma acted like a foreign body. Patients failed to fully react to a trauma. They claimed that the splitting of consciousness described in dual personality happened in every hysteria. However, hidden memories were retrievable under hypnosis. Each hysterical symptom disappeared when one succeeded in bringing to light the memory of the event which provoked it, and the patient had put the affect into words. The psychical processes had to be brought back 'in statu nascendi'. They famously concluded that, 'Hysterics suffer mainly from reminiscences.'[37] After the collapse of Freud's so-called seduction theory and his abandonment of hypnosis, the therapeutic emphasis no longer focussed on rememoration and catharsis, but on the interpretation of and working through of Oedipal fantasies by way of free association, dream analysis, and transference interpretation.

In the psychoanalytic and psychotherapeutic literature, 'interpretation' increasingly came to take the preeminent place previously occupied by 'suggestion'. Jacqueline Carroy has noted that in the hypnotic literature, suggestion functioned as a heterodox, umbrella term, which, as well as imperative suggestion, included paradoxical injunctions and interpretations.[38] In a similar manner, if one studies psychoanalytic and psychotherapeutic cases in the twentieth century, one finds that 'interpretation' functioned in a similar catch-all manner. Whilst the theoretical account of practices changed considerably, the same was not the case in the practices themselves, and under the rubric of interpretation in the psychoanalytic literature, it is not hard to find some of the best examples of authoritarian directives.

It was with the entrance of Bleuler (1857–1939), Jung (1875–1961), and the Zürich school that the psychoanalytic movement truly become international. It was Bleuler and Jung that put psychoanalysis on the map in the German-speaking psychiatric world. The ease with which individuals could gain instruction in psychoanalytic techniques in the Burghölzli was similar to Bernheim's clinic in Nancy, and led greatly to their dissemination. Indeed, for psychiatrists interested in psychoanalysis, Zürich, and not Vienna, was initially the instruction centre of choice. As Ernst Falzeder notes, a large proportion of significant figures in dynamic psychiatry and psychoanalysis either worked or visited the Burghölzli.[39] The open model of instruction practised there greatly contributed to the spread of psychoanalysis. However, it quickly came into collision with the closed feudal structure which Freud was establishing.

In 1909, August Forel (1848–1931), a major champion of hypnosis and suggestion, founded the International Society for Medical Psychology and Psychotherapy. In August, he sent circulars off to the principal representatives of European psychotherapy, including Freud and Jung, asking them to join. Forel felt that the lack of coordination between different orientations in psychotherapy was a critical problem. He wanted to create order in this 'Tower of Babel' by facilitating scientific exchanges and establishing 'a clear international terminology, capable of being accepted in a general manner by different people'[40] – in other words, to form one general science of psychotherapy. Shortly after, Freud proposed the idea of a rival association of psychoanalysis, firmly grouping together adherents to his doctrine. This timing was not accidental.[41]

Freud contended that psychoanalytic technique could as yet not be learnt from books, but only from someone already proficient in it. Due to the dangers of 'wild' psychoanalysis, he and his co-workers had founded the International Psycho-Analytic Association.[42] Freud was militantly opposed to psychoanalysis freely entering general medical practice as an auxiliary psychotherapeutic procedure – not out of some concern with safeguarding the public, but with safeguarding psychoanalysis and the purity of the doctrine. Indeed, it was due to the increasing isolationist policy of psychoanalysis *vis-à-vis* medicine and psychiatry that Eugen Bleuler resigned from the

IPA in 1911.[43] It was Freud's institutional model rather than Forel's that came to predominate in the twentieth century.

In 1912, Jung put forward the recommendation that every prospective analyst had to undergo an analysis, arguing that success in analysis depended upon how far the analyst had been analysed himself.[44] Jung's suggestion was quickly seconded by Freud. It was insufficient simply to be a doctor or psychiatrist to practise psychoanalysis. Whilst claiming that psychoanalysis was a medical technique, further qualification was required. In terms of current practices in psychotherapy, this was a striking departure. It would have been unthinkable to have established the hypnotic treatment of the physician as an essential training requirement. Freud argued that the would-be analyst had to undergo a 'psycho-analytic purification'.[45] The training analysis was the means by which the faithful transmission of analytic knowledge was safeguarded.

Jung's suggestion has had an overpowering effect, not only on the subsequent organisation of psychoanalysis, but on modern psychotherapy. Until recently, this requirement has been one of the few common denominators in the plethora of psychotherapeutic schools. The institution of training analysis became critical in providing a financial base for private practice psychoanalysis and helped to make it a viable professional proposition.

After the hiatus of the Second World War, the institutionalisation of the psychoanalytic movement spread place rapidly.[46] The Berlin society, founded by Karl Abraham in 1920, began to formalise its training. It was here that the triad of personal analysis, supervised analysis, and seminars was established that became the basic template of all psychoanalytic institutes. In 1925, at the psychoanalytic congress in Bad Homburg, the stipulation the requirement that every prospective analyst had to be analysed was passed.

It was through the training enterprise that psychoanalysis prospered from the 1920s onwards. The formation of a psychoanalytic training system, detached from medicine and psychiatry was crucial in the survival of psychoanalysis, and greatly contributed to its success in comparison with other forms of psychotherapy, as no other school had established a comparable system. The public success of psychoanalysis was not due to any inherent therapeutic or theoretical superiority, but from the particular mode of institutional organisation that it adopted and the consequent suggestive effect on the wider populace. Without this, the Freudian legend would have been ineffective. It was the effectiveness of the institutional structures of psychoanalysis that gave it public visibility, such that cultural debates about the new psychology were nominally cast in the idiom of psychoanalysis.

If the establishment of the psychoanalytic training system played a crucial role in the establishment of psychoanalysis, it was also an unstable matrix, as it could easily become adapted to any theoretical model. This has indeed been the case, and a myriad of psychotherapeutic schools adopted the same institutional structure to propagate their therapies. The success of these rival schools, adopting the same institutional structures as psychoanalysis, contributed to the decline of psychoanalysis.

In addition to being a psychotherapeutic procedure, Freud extended the scope of psychoanalysis to the analysis and diagnosis of culture in general, in such works as *Civilisation and its Discontents* and *The Future of an Illusion*.[47] Freud's expansion of the neurosis concept in works such as *The Psychopathology of Everyday Life*,[48] and his pathologisation of culture, led to an implicit conception that the freedom from neurosis promised by psychoanalytic therapy constituted, if not a state of well-being, a lesser state of ill-being than of a large proportion of the population. The patient pool for psychoanalytic therapy had in effect been extended to everyone.

A similar expansion took place in the work of Jung, in a radically different and more melioristic manner. In 1913, Jung had a series of apocalyptic visions. Struck by the correspondence between these and the subsequent onset of the war, Jung engaged in a process of self-experimentation which he termed his 'confrontation with the unconscious'. At the heart of this project was Jung's attempt to get to know his own 'myth' as a solution to the mythless predicament of secular modernity. This took the form of provoking an extended series of waking fantasies in himself. Jung elaborated, illustrated, and commented on these fantasies in a work that he called *Liber Novus*, or *The Red Book*, which was at the centre of his later work.[49] This depicted the process through which Jung regained his soul and overcame the contemporary malaise of spiritual alienation, which was achieved through enabling the rebirth of a new image of God in his soul and developing a new world view in the form of a psychological and theological cosmology. *Liber Novus* presented the prototype of Jung's conception of the individuation process, which he held to be the universal form of individual psychological development.

In 1916, Jung wrote a paper on 'The Transcendent Function', developing a generalisable psychotherapeutic method from his self-experimentation. He later termed this 'active imagination'. One commenced by concentrating on a particular mood and attempting to become as conscious as possible of all fantasies and associations which came up in connection with it. The aim was to allow fantasy free play, but without departing from the initial affect in a free associative process. This led to a concrete or symbolic expression of the mood, which had the result of bringing the affect nearer to consciousness, hence making it more understandable. The mere process of doing this could have a vitalising effect. Individuals could write, draw, paint or sculpt, depending on their propensities.[50] Once these fantasies had been produced and embodied, two approaches were possible: creative formulation and understanding. Each needed the other, and both were necessary to produce the transcendent function, which arose out of the union of conscious and unconscious contents, and resulted in a widening of consciousness. In his practice at this time, Jung encouraged his patients to undertake similar forms of self-investigation. His use and advocacy of nonverbal techniques in psychotherapy was to play an important role in the rise of art therapies.[51]

Jung maintained that his fantasies and those of his patients stemmed from the mythopoetic imagination which was missing in the present rational age. Reconnecting with this could form the basis for cultural renewal. The task of moderns was one of establishing a dialogue with the contents of the collective unconscious and integrating them into consciousness. This was to play an important part in the popular 'mythic revival'. He maintained that cultural renewal could only come about through self-regeneration of the individual; in other words, through the individuation process. Consequently, for Jung psychotherapy was no longer a process solely preoccupied with the treatment of psychopathology. It became a practice to enable the higher development of the individual through fostering individuation. Jung noted that a third of his cases had no neurosis, and were highly functioning and well-adapted individuals, but who had an acute sense of aimlessness.[52] The task that they confronted was that of a recovery of a sense of meaning in their life, made more pressing with the secularisation and rationalisation of contemporary culture. Thus such individuals were suffering from a condition that afflicted the culture at large. Consequently, individuals who managed to recover a sense of meaning in their lives were healing not only themselves, but also the culture. This broadening of the aims of psychotherapy to encompass the higher, spiritual development of the individual played an important role in the rise of humanistic and transpersonal psychologies and psychotherapies, and soul therapies.[53]

Shellshock during the First World War had led to an increasing recognition of the prevalence of purely psychic disorders and legitimacy of psychic treatment. Correspondingly, the expansion of the neurosis concept was linked with an increasing destigmatisation. During the 1920s and 1930s, psychotherapy was dominated, on the one hand, by the still-widespread, eclectic use of hypnosis and suggestion, and on the other, by the work of figures such as Janet, Freud, Jung, and Adler, in which conceptions of psychotherapy were tightly linked to proprietary systems of dynamic psychology. Bernheim's ontology of suggestion was a relatively sparse and simple one. By contrast the ontologies of the unconscious on offer in Freudian and Jungian therapies were vast baroque structures that generated some of the most complex hermeneutic systems of the twentieth century.[54] They took hold in the humanities and social sciences and also had powerful effects on the wider populace, furnishing compelling forms of self-description and other-ascription.

After Freud, there was also a shift in psychoanalysis to more melioristic conceptions of the aims and possibilities of psychoanalytic therapy. For example, in her work, *Neurosis and Human Growth: The Struggle Toward Self Realization* (1951), Karen Horney (1885–1952) tried to shift psychoanalysis away from a medical model, arguing instead that it was a practice that fostered self-realisation. Its aim was one of aiding an individual to outgrow difficulties so that their development 'may assume a more constructive course' through releasing innate healing forces and mobilising the real self.[55] As a consequence, analysis came to be seen to be following in the footsteps of distinguished forebears: 'The road of analytic therapy is an old one, advocated time and again throughout human history. In the terms of Socrates and the Hindu philosophy, among others, it is the *road to reorientation through self-knowledge.*'[56] Self-realisation, in turn, was now depicted in a psychological idiom, consisting in a deeper experiencing of one's feelings, wishes and beliefs, the ability to use one's resources, a greater sense of responsibility, relating to others with genuine feelings, respecting them as individuals in a spirit of mutuality, becoming more productive, and valuing work intrinsically, rather than as a means to satisfy pride and vanity. The result of this was facilitating the desire for and the possibility of happiness.[57] Throughout Horney's work, there was a clear alignment of the goals of therapy with dominant cultural norms.

The 1940s and 1950s saw the rise of systems of psychotherapy no longer tightly linked with general systems of psychology, such as the humanistic psychotherapy, or the 'client-centered therapy', promulgated by Carl Rogers (1902–1987). In 1951, Rogers argued that in client-centered therapy there was no need for theories without phenomena to explain in the form of observable changes.[58] In place of top-down theory dominated psychotherapies, Rogers advocated what one could call 'theory-lite' psychotherapies, legitimated by the study of process notes and outcomes. Under Rogers' ministrations, psychotherapy led to certain characteristic changes of behaviour: an increased discussion of plans and behavioral steps to be undertaken while in therapy; a change from relatively immature to mature behaviour; a decrease in psychological tension and defensive behaviours coupled with greater awareness of those defensive behaviours which are present; an increased tolerance for frustration as objectively measured in physiological terms; and improved functioning in life tasks and in adjustment to job training and job performance.[59] The successful clients of Rogers's therapy – a term popularised in his 1942 study[60] – were clearly intended to take up their role as good citizens in advanced liberal democratic societies. For Rogers, they would not necessarily be adjusted to the culture, nor be conformists, but would live constructively and be in sync with their culture to the extent required by a balanced satisfaction of needs. As a result, they would be vanguards of human evolution.[61] Rogers in turn attributed the rise of psychotherapy to societal transformations, and in particular, to the manner in which, as culture became less homogenous, it gave less support to individuals, who consequently could no longer rely on culture and tradition. Hence individuals needed to resolve in themselves issues previously determined by society. As it offered a means of resolving such conflicts, psychotherapy had increasingly become a public and professional focal point.[62]

Rogers's work is an example of the malleability of psychotherapy, with regard to determination of the changes deemed beneficial and held to be therapeutic in a particular social epoch, and one resting on a particular 'image of man', which it in turn helped to promote: 'The basic nature of the human being, when functioning freely, is constructive and trustworthy.'[63] This was presented as an alternative to Freud's mordant, tragic vision.

The rise of the psychotherapies also played a significant factor in the development of what cultural historians have called the 'therapeutic ethos'. Jackson Lears has argued that the first decades of the twentieth century in America were marked by a crucial moral change from 'a Protestant ethos of salvation through self-denial toward a therapeutic ethos stressing self-realization in this world'.[64] This therapeutic ethos was in turn taken up and reinforced by advertisers, who attempted to respond to and shape the emotional needs of consumers. This led to the presentation of products as embodiments of the therapeutic ethos. As Lears puts it, 'the promise was that the product would contribute to the buyer's physical, psychic, or social well-being; and the threat was that his well-being would be undermined if he failed to buy it.'[65] In this way the therapeutic ethos was a critical constituent of mass consumer culture. Consequently, psychotherapies were having far-ranging effects beyond therapists' consulting rooms.

The same period saw the rise of the existential psychotherapies, predicated on a different 'image of man'. Existential therapists articulated cultural critiques, coupled with critiques of the role of psychotherapies in contributing to the modern malaise of social alienation. In his contribution to the volume that did much to popularise existential therapies in the English-speaking world, *Existence*, Rollo May argued that 'the fundamental neurotic process in our day is the repression of the ontological sense.'[66] This resulted in a truncation of awareness and loss of innate potentialities. The diagnosis for the problems afflicting moderns was to be found in Heidegger's *Being and Time*. For May, practised in an unreflective manner, psychotherapy could simply serve to make matters worse by simply reflecting 'the fragmentation of the culture', and hence 'structuralizing neurosis rather than curing it'.[67] The fact that patients came to psychotherapy aiming to be cured from neurotic symptoms was itself the problem, which therapists should not collude in. The 'promise' that psychotherapies were offering of curing pathology – of conceiving the problems of existence in quasi-medical terms – was actually making things worse. By contrast, May argued that therapy should be concerned with enabling an individual to experience their existence. Any relief of symptoms which arose would be a by-product of this. The ideal of 'cure' conceived of as adjustment and fitting in with culture could be brought about through technically conceived therapies, as contemporary culture mandated living in a calculated well-managed manner. Such practices would lead to a lessening of anxiety, through a curtailment of the freedom which gave rise to anxiety, but this only resulted in a constriction of one's existence. Psychotherapists had become agents of the culture, and the practice of psychotherapy had become an expression of contemporary fragmentation, rather than a solution to it. Sartre, Heidegger, and Kierkegaard were now mobilised and operationalised into psychotherapeutic discourse.

Cultural critique took an explicit form in Gestalt therapy. In 1951, Frederick Perls (1893–1970), Ralph Hefferline (1910–1974), and Paul Goodman (1911–1972) argued that in contrast to other therapies, Gestalt therapy focussed on the actual situation, rather than viewing it as a symptom or as an expression of some unconscious content.[68] They were directly challenging prevailing value systems in psychotherapy, proposing a transvaluation of values, such as 'infantile' and 'mature'. The personalities of psychotherapists and their social role had led to the championing of the latter over the former: devaluing childhood traits and promoting adaptation to 'a standard of adult reality that is not worth adjusting to'.[69] In place of conformity to the so-called 'reality principle', they championed creative adjustment, arguing that the former consisted of social illusions that cast creative spontaneity as dangerous or psychotic.[70] Gestalt therapy aligned itself with the burgeoning counter-culture.

Meanwhile, other forms of psychotherapy arose which presented themselves as more culturally syntonic. In his landmark *Cognitive Therapy and the Emotional Disorders* of 1976, Aaron Beck (1921–), an American psychiatrist and psychoanalyst presented the following 'Formula for treatment': 'The therapist helps a patient to unravel his distortions in thinking and to learn alternative, more realistic ways to formulate his experiences.'[71] No reader of Paul Dubois can read this without a sense of déjà vu, nor fail to see cognitive therapy as a revival of a revival of moral treatment. Pinel is truly back. Beck quite consciously viewed cognitive therapy as the promotion of a new 'image of man':

> This new approach to emotional disorders changes man's perspective on himself and his problems. Rather than viewing himself as the helpless creature of his own biochemical reactions, or of blind impulses, or of automatic reflexes, he can regard himself as prone to learning erroneous, self-defeating notions and capable of *unlearning* or correcting them as well.[72]

What is on offer here is, in effect, a new optional ontology: one that can be characterised as 'therapeutic rationality'. In 'therapeutic rationality', disordered thought is the pathogen, and regulation of thought is the cure. Rachel Rosner has recently demonstrated that far from being an alternative to psychoanalysis, Beck conceived of cognitive therapy as a branch of neo-Freudianism.[73] For Beck, cognitive therapy had the advantages of psychoanalysis, without the drawbacks. Critically, it was readily amenable to experimental testing and easily accomodatable to the protocols of evidence-based medicine. Compared to psychoanalysis, the ontology on offer in cognitive therapy is a radically stripped down one – gone are all the denizens of the inner world and their metapsychological doubles. Cognitive therapy represents a new minimalism of the mind. Critically, gone too was the elaborate, lengthy, and costly apprenticeship system of psychoanalytic and psychotherapeutic training, and with it, the essential requirement that a would-be practitioner was required to undergo an initiatory treatment themselves, to experience the practice at first hand. This shift in mode of instruction has enabled the mass rollout of state-funded cognitive behaviour therapy in the UK, to take one example.[74]

As Delboeuf had pointed out with regard to hypnosis, the cultural dissemination of psychotherapeutic ideas in turn shaped the patients who came to psychotherapy, leading to a Moebius strip of circulating feedback loops. By the mid-twentieth century, the psychotherapeutic scene was a teeming marketplace, offering a plethora of competing optional ontologies: conceptions not only of the reasons for one's maladies and how to be cured of them, but of how to be well and take up one's place in society and the world. These were not only illness narratives in Arthur Kleinman's sense,[75] but also what one could call transformation narratives. Psychotherapy had become not only a palliative for psychological disorders, but a form of life enhancement. As such, it increasingly became a lifestyle choice. The varieties of psychotherapy on offer constituted choices of various regimens of well-being, of achieving, in the Aristotelian sense, the good life. The conceptions of well-being on offer were seen to be legitimated by, if not science, something close to it, with the same universalistic aspirations.

Thus, psychotherapies have played critical roles in fostering conceptions of psychological disorder as well as of psychological well-being and identity itself. Since psychotherapy began to gain increasing currency towards the end of the nineteenth century, it and its surrounding cultures have both undergone mutations and transformations, acting on and reacting to one another in a series of relations, at times in concert, at times antagonistically. We have yet to comprehend the full scale of its effects on contemporary societies which have, in part, become psychotherapeutic societies. It was not for nothing that that Marshall McLuhan stated in 1964, 'ours is the century of the psychiatrist's couch.'[76]

Notes

1 Frederick van Eeden, 'Les principes de la psychothérapie', *Revue de l'hypnotisme*, 7 (1893): 99. Van Eeden had founded a 'clinique de psycho-thérapeutique suggestive' in 1889 with Albert van Rentergehm.

2 Karl Jaspers, *General Psychopathology*, tr. J. Hoening and Marian Hamilton (Manchester: Manchester University Press, 1963), 834.

3 Thomas Szasz, 'The Myth of Psychotherapy', *Proceedings of the 9th International Congress of Psychotherapy, Oslo, 1973* (Basel: S. Karger, 1975), 220.

4 This was presented in a series of linked neologisms: 'Psychogenesis – the birth of thought/ psychophrenologia – the home of thought/psychopathia – the bane of thought/ psychotherapeia – the antidote of thought/psychonoesis – the force of thought.' See the table of contents in Walter Cooper Dendy, *Psyche: A Discourse on the Birth and Pilgrimage of Thought* (London: Longman, Brown, Green and Longmans, 1853).

5 Dendy, 'Psychotherapeia, or the Remedial Influence of Mind', *Journal of Psychological Medicine and Mental Pathology*, 6 (1853): 268.
6 *Asylum Journal*, 8 (1854): 127.
7 D. H. Tuke, *Illustrations of the Influence of the Mind Upon the Body in Health and Disease Designed to Elucidate the Action of the Imagination* (London: J. & A. Churchill, 1872). The next few pages draw from my '"Psychotherapy": The Invention of a Word', *History of the Human Sciences*, 18 (2005): 1–25, in a revised and modified form.
8 Ibid., 405. Tuke was referring to *Report of Dr. Benjamin Franklin and other commissioners charged by the King of France with the examination of the animal magnetism, as now practised at Paris*, tr. William Goodwin (London: J. Johnson, 1785).
9 Ibid., 5.
10 Hippolyte Bernheim, *Bernheim's New Studies in Hypnotism* [Hypnotisme, suggestion, psycho-thérapie: études nouvelles, 1891], tr. R. Sandor (New York: International Universities Press, 1980), 16.
11 Ibid., 18.
12 Bernheim, in Tuke ed., *A Dictionary of Psychological Medicine* (London: J. A. Churchill, 1892), 1214.
13 Henrik Petersen, 'Hypno-suggestion, etc., Medical letters' in Otto Wetterstrand, *Hypnotism and its Application to Practical Medicine*, tr. Petersen (New York: G. P. Putnam, 1897), 126.
14 Jean-Martin Charcot, *Clinical Lectures on the Diseases of the Nervous System*, ed. Ruth Harris (London: Routledge, 1991).
15 Joseph Delboeuf, 'De l'influence de l'education et de l'imitation dans le somnambulisme provoqué', *Revue Philosophique*, 22 (1886): 52–3.
16 Tuke, *Le corps et l'esprit. Action du moral et de l'imagination sur le physique*, tr. V. Parent (Paris: J.-B. Ballière, 1886).
17 Bernheim, *De la suggestion et de ses applications à la thérapeutique* (Paris: Doin, 1886), 218.
18 Delboeuf, 'Quelques considérations sur la psychologie de l'hypnotisme, à propos d'un cas de manie homicide guérie par suggestion', (1893), in *Le Sommeil et les rêves et autres textes* (Paris: Fayard, 1993), 421.
19 Paul Dubois, *Psychic Treatment of Nervous Disorders* [*Les Psychonévroses et leur traitement moral*] (1904), tr. S. E. Jeliffe and W. A. White (New York: Funk & Wagnalls, 1909), 221.
20 Ibid., xiii.
21 Ibid., 96.
22 A similar perspective was presented by Jules Déjerine and E. Glaucker, *The Psychoneuroses and their Treatment by Psychotherapy* (1911) [*Les manifestations fonctionnelles des psychonévroses: leur traitement par la psychothérapie*], tr. S. E. Jelliffe (Philadelphia, PA: J. B. Lippincott, 1918). On this question, see Marcel Gauchet and Gladys Swain, 'Du traitement moral aux psychothérapies: remarque sur la formation de l'idée contemporaine de psychothérapie', in Gladys Swain, *Dialogues avec l'insensé* (Paris: Gallimard, 1994), 237–262.
23 Dubois, *Les psychonévroses et leur traitement moral*, (Paris: Masson, 1905, 2nd edn), 19.
24 On this question, see Mikkel Borch-Jacobsen, *Making Minds and Madness: From Hysteria to Depression* (Cambridge: Cambridge University Press, 2009), and my 'Claire, Lise, Jean, Nadia, and Gisèle: Preliminary Notes towards a Characterisation of Pierre Janet's Psychasthenia' in *Cultures of Neurasthenia: From Beard to the First World War*, ed. Marijke Gijswijt-Hofstra and Roy Porter (Amsterdam: Rodopi, 2001), 362–385.
25 Jean Camus and Philippe Pagniez, *Isolement et psychothérapie: traitement de l'hystérie et de la neurasthénie, pratique de la rééducation morale et physique* (Paris: Alcan, 1904), 26.
26 See Sanjay Subrahmanyam, *Explorations in Connected History: From the Tagus to the Ganges* (Delhi: Oxford University Press, 2004).
27 On this issue, see my 'Psychologies as Ontology-Making Practices: William James and the Pluralities of Psychological Experience' in *William James and the Varieties of Religious Experience*, ed. Jeremy Carrette, (London: Routledge, 2004), 27–46.
28 Pierre Janet, *L'Automatisme psychologique: essais de psychologie expérimentale sur les formes inférieures de l'activité humaine*, 4th edition (Paris: Alcan, 1903).
29 Pierre Janet, *Mental State of Hystericals: A Study of Mental Stigmata and Mental Accidents*, tr. C. Corson (New York: G. P. Putnam's Sons, 1901).

30 Pierre Janet, *Les obsessions et la psychasthénie* I (Paris: Alcan, 1903), 727.
31 See for instance Elwood Worcester, Samuel McComb and Isador Coriat, *Religion and Medicine: The Moral Control of Nervous Disorders* (New York: Moffat Yard, 1908). See Eric Caplan, *Mind Games: American Culture and the Birth of Psychotherapy* (Berkeley, CA: University of California Press, 2001).
32 Pierre Janet, *Psychological Healing*, tr. E & C Paul, (London: Allen & Unwin, 1925).
33 See for example, Henri Ellenberger, *The Discovery of the Unconscious: The History and Evolution of Dynamic Psychiatry* (New York: Basic Books, 1970).
34 Ibid., 1208.
35 See Frank Sulloway, *Freud, Biologist of the Mind: Beyond the Psychoanalytic Legend*, (Cambridge, MA: Harvard University Press, 1992) and Mikkel Borch-Jacobsen and Sonu Shamdasani, *The Freud Files: An Inquiry into the History of Psychoanalysis*, (Cambridge: Cambridge University Press, 2012).
36 Josef Breuer and Sigmund Freud, 'On the Psychical Mechanism of Hysteria: Preliminary Communication,' *The Standard Edition of the Complete Psychological Works of Sigmund Freud*, ed. James Strachey, Anna Freud, Alix Strachey, Alan Tyson and Angela Richards (London: Hogarth Press and the Institute of Psycho-Analysis, 1953–1974). (Hereafter, SE), vol. 2.
37 Ibid., 10.
38 Jacqueline Carroy, *Hypnose, suggestion et psychologie: l'invention de sujets* (Paris: PUF, 1991), 179–200.
39 Ernst Falzeder, 'The Threads of Psychoanalytic Filiations or Psychoanalysis Taking Effect', in *100 Years of Psychoanalysis: Contributions to the History of Psychoanalysis*, ed. André Haynal and Ernst Falzeder, special issue of *Cahiers Psychiatriques Genevois* 1994, 172.
40 August Forel, 'La psychologie et la psychothérapie à l'université', *Journal für Psychologie und Neurologie*, 17 (1910): 315–316.
41 See Mikkel Borch-Jacobsen and Sonu Shamdasani, *The Freud Files: An Inquiry into the History of Psychoanalysis* (Cambridge: Cambridge University Press), 77f., and my '"Psychotherapy in 1909: Notes on a Vintage', in *After Freud Left: New Reflections on a Century of Psychoanalysis in America*, ed. John Burnham (Chicago: University of Chicago Press, 2012), 31–47.
42 Freud, '"Wild" Psycho-analysis', *SE* 11, 226–227.
43 Bleuler to Freud, in Eugen Bleuler and Sigmund Freud, *'Ich bin zuversichtlich, wir erobern bald die Psychiatrie.' Briefwechsel 1904–1937*, ed, Michael Schröter (Basel: Schwabe, 2012), 153f. See Ernst Falzeder, 'The Story of an Ambivalent Relationship: Sigmund Freud and Eugen Bleuler', *Journal of Analytical Psychology*, 52 (2007): 343–368.
44 Jung, 'Attempt at a Portrayal of Psychoanalytic Theory', *Collected Works*, 4, ed. Gerhard Adler, Michael Fordham, Herbert Read, William McGuire, tr. R. F. C. Hull, (New York and Princeton: Bollingen Series and London, 1953–1983), (hereafter, *CW*) vol. 4, section 449.
45 Freud, 'Recommendations to Physicians Practising Psycho-analysis', (1912) *SE* 12, 116.
46 See Ernst Falzeder, *Psychoanalytic Filiations: Mapping the Psychoanalytic Movement* (London: Karnac, 2015) and George Makari, *Revolution in Mind: The Creation of Psychoanalysis* (New York: HarperCollins, 2008).
47 Freud, *SE* 21.
48 Freud, *SE* 6.
49 Jung, *The Red Book. Liber Novus*, ed. Sonu Shamdasani, trs. Mark Kyburz, John Peck and Sonu Shamdasani (New York: W. W. Norton, 2009).
50 Jung, *CW* 8, sections 170–171.
51 See Susan Hogan, *Healing Arts: The History of Art Therapy* (London: Jessica Kingsley, 2001).
52 'The Aims of Psychotherapy' (1929), *CW* 6, § 83.
53 See Eugene Taylor, *Shadow Culture: Psychology and Spirituality in America* (Washington, DC: Counterpoint, 1999).
54 See my 'The Optional Unconscious' in *Thinking the Unconscious: Nineteenth-Century German Thought*, ed. Martin Liebscher and Angus Nicholls (Cambridge: Cambridge University Press, 2010), 287–296.
55 Karen Horney, *Neurosis and Human Growth: the Struggle Toward Self Realization* (New York: W. W. Norton, 1951), 33.
56 Ibid., 341.

57 Karen Horney, *New Ways in Psychoanalysis* (London: Kegan Paul, Trench and Trubner, 1947), 290.
58 Carl Rogers, *Client-Centered Therapy: Its Current Practice, Implications and Theory* (Boston: Houghton Mifflin Co., 1951), 15.
59 Ibid., 179f.
60 Carl Rogers, *Counselling and Psychotherapy* (New York: Houghton, Mifflin & Co, 1942).
61 Carl Rogers, *On Becoming a Person: A Therapist's View of Psychotherapy* (London: John Constable, 1961), 191f.
62 Carl Rogers, *Client-Centered Therapy: Its Current Practice, Implications and Theory*, 4.
63 Carl Rogers, *On Becoming a Person: A Therapist's View of Psychotherapy*, 194.
64 T. J. Jackson Lears, "From Salvation to Self-Realization: Advertising and the Therapeutic Roots of the Consumer Culture, 1880–1930," *Advertising & Society Review*, 1 (2000), E-ISSSN, section 4.
65 Ibid., 50.
66 Rollo May, 'Contributions of Existential Psychotherapy' in *Existence: A New Dimension in Psychology and Psychiatry*, ed. Rollo May, Ernest Angel and Henri Ellenberger (New York: Basic Books, 1958), 86.
67 Ibid., 86–7.
68 Frederick Perls, Ralph Hefferline and Paul Goodman, et al., *Gestalt therapy: Excitement and Growth in the Human Personality* (New York: Julian Press, 1951), 237.
69 Ibid., 241.
70 Ibid., 394.
71 Aaron Beck, *Cognitive Therapy and the Emotional Disorders* (New York: International Universities Press, 1976), 3.
72 Ibid., 4.
73 Rachel Rosner, 'The "Splendid Isolation" of Aaron T. Beck', *Isis* 105 (2014): 736.
74 See Richard Layard and David Clark, *Thrive: The Power of Evidence-Based Psychological Therapies* (London: Penguin, 2014). On the history of cognitive behaviour therapy, see Sarah Marks, 'Cognitive Behaviour Therapies in Britain: The Historical Context and Present Situation', in *Cognitive Behaviour Therapies*, ed. Windy Dryden, (London: Sage, 2012), 1–25.
75 Arthur Kleinman, *The Illness Narratives: Suffering Healing, and the Human Condition* (New York: Basic Books, 1988).
76 Marshall McLuhan, *Understanding Media: The Extensions of Man* (New York: McGraw Hill, 1964), 7.

Suggestion, persuasion and work: Psychotherapies in communist Europe

Sarah Marks

ABSTRACT

This article traces what recent research and primary sources tell us about psychotherapy in Communist Europe, and how it survived both underground and above the surface. In particular, I will elaborate on the psychotherapeutic techniques that were popular across the different countries and language cultures of the Soviet sphere, with a particular focus upon the Cold War period. This article examines the literature on the mixed fortunes of psychoanalysis and group therapies in the region. More specifically, it focuses upon the therapeutic modalities such as work therapy, suggestion and rational therapy, which gained particular popularity in the Communist countries of Central and Eastern Europe. The latter two approaches had striking similarities with parallel developments in behavioural and cognitive therapies in the West. In part, this was because clinicians on both sides of the 'iron curtain' drew upon shared European traditions from the late nineteenth and early twentieth centuries. Nevertheless, this article argues that in the Soviet sphere, those promoting these approaches appropriated socialist thought as a source of inspiration and justification, or at the very least, as a convenient political shield.

EL TRABAJO DE LA SUGESTION Y LA PERSUACION: psicoterapias en la Europa comunista- Marks:

Este artículo rastrea lo que las investigaciones recientes y fuentes fidedignas nos dicen acerca de la psicoterapia en la Europa comunista y cómo ésta sobrevivió en dos formas: abiertamente y en la clandestinidad. Particularmente me referiré a las técnicas psicoterapéuticas que fueron populares a través de los diferentes países y lenguajes culturales de la esfera soviética con especial foco en el período de la "guerra fria". Se examina la literatura acerca de la suerte desigual del psicoanálisis y de las terapias de grupo en la región, concentrándonos específicamente en algunas modalidades como la terapia de trabajo, la sugestión y la terapia racional, las cuales fueron muy utilizadas en los países comunistas de la Europa Central y del Este. Los últimos dos métodos tuvieron sorprendentes similitudes con el desarrollo de la terapia behaviorista y las terapias cognitivas en el Oeste. De alguna manera ésto fue así, porque a ambos lados de la "cortina de hierro" los profesionales se inspiraron en las tradiciones europeas compartidas desde finales del siglo XIX y principios del siglo XX; sin embargo, este artículo argumenta que dentro de la esfera soviética aquéllos que promovieron estos métodos se apropiaron del pensamiento socialista como fuente de inspiración y justificación o al menos como un escudo político conveniente.

Suggestione, persuasione e lavoro: psicoterapie nell'Europa comunista- Marks

Questo articolo tratteggia ciò che la ricerca recente e le fonti principali dicono della psicoterapia nell'Europa comunista e di come essa sia sopravvissuta sia in modo nascosto sia in modo più evidente. Inoltre, vengono approfondite le tecniche psicoterapeutiche più popolari nei diversi paesi e culture della sfera sovietica, con particolare attenzione al periodo della Guerra Fredda. L'articolo esamina quindi la letteratura sulle fortune alterne della psicoanalisi e delle terapie di gruppo in questa area geografica. Più specificamente, si focalizza su alcune prassi terapeutiche come la terapia del lavoro, la suggestione e la terapia razionale che hanno avuto ampia popolarità nei paesi comunisti dell'Europa centrale e orientale. Gli ultimi due approcci presentano sorprendenti somiglianze con le terapie comportamentali e cognitive che, in parallelo, si andavano sviluppando in Occidente. Ciò era anche dovuto al fatto che i clinici di entrambe le parti della "cortina di ferro" attingevano da tradizioni europee condivise tra la fine del XIX e l'inizio del XX secolo. Tuttavia, questo articolo sostiene che nella sfera sovietica, coloro che promuovevano questi approcci si appropriavano del pensiero socialista come fonte di ispirazione e giustificazione, o per lo meno come un conveniente scudo politico.

Suggestion, persuasion et travail: psychothérapies dans l'Europe communiste - Marks

Cet article retrace ce que les recherches récentes et les sources principales nous disent au sujet de la psychothérapie dans l'Europe communiste et comment elle a survécu à la fois de manière souterraine et en surface. Je mettrai l'accent, en particulier, sur les techniques psychothérapeutiques qui étaient populaires dans les différents pays et cultures langagières de la sphère soviétique avec une référence plus spécifique à la période de la guerre froide. Cet article examine la littérature portant sur les résultats mitigés de la psychanalyse et des thérapies de groupe dans cette région. Il se concentre plus spécifiquement sur les modalités thérapeutiques telles que la thérapie par le travail, la suggestion et la thérapie rationnelle, qui furent très populaires dans les pays communistes d'Europe Centrale et de l'Est. Les deux dernières modalités présentent des ressemblances étonnantes avec les développements des thérapies comportementales et cognitives de l'Ouest. Ceci est dû en partie au fait que les cliniciens des deux côtés du rideau de fer se sont inspirés de traditions européennes communes datant de la fin du 19ieme, début du 20ieme siècle. Cependant cet article soutient que dans la sphère soviétique, ceux qui promouvaient ces approches s'appropriaient la pensée socialiste en tant que source d'inspiration et de justification, ou tout du moins, en faisait le bouclier politique idéal.

Υποβολή, πειθώ και εργασία»: Η ψυχοθεραπεία στην κομμουνιστική Ευρώπη- Sarah Marks

Περίληψη: Αυτό το άρθρο εστιάζει στις πρόσφατες έρευνες και στις πρωταρχικές πηγές για την ψυχοθεραπεία στην Κομμουνιστική Ευρώπη και το πώς επιβίωσε τόσο κάτω όσο και πάνω από την επιφάνεια. Συγκεκριμένα, θα αναπτύξω τις ψυχοθεραπευτικές τεχνικές που ήταν δημοφιλείς στις διαφορετικές χώρες και γλωσσικές κουλτούρες που βρισκόταν κάτω από τη σφαίρα επιρροής της Σοβιετικής Ένωσης, με ιδιαίτερη εστίαση στην περίοδο του Ψυχρού Πολέμου. Αυτό το άρθρο εξετάζει την βιβλιογραφία που αφορά την ανάμικτη μοίρα που είχε η ψυχανάλυση και η ομαδική θεραπεία σε αυτές τις περιοχές. Πιο συγκεκριμένα, εστιάζει σε θεραπευτικές πρακτικές όπως είναι η θεραπεία μέσω εργασίας, η θεραπεία βάσει υποβολής και λογικής, που έγιναν ιδιαίτερα δημοφιλείς στις Κομμουνιστικές χώρες της Κεντρικής Ανατολικής Ευρώπης. Οι δύο τελευταίες προσεγγίσεις είχαν εντυπωσιακές ομοιότητες με την παράλληλη ανάπτυξη των συμπεριφορικών και γνωστικών θεραπειών στη Δύση. Εν μέρει, αυτό συνέβη γιατί οι κλινικοί και στις δύο πλευρές του «σιδηρούντος παραπετάσματος» άντλησαν από κοινές ευρωπαϊκές παραδόσεις από τα τέλη του 19ου και τις αρχές του 20ου αιώνα. Ωστόσο, το παρόν άρθρο υποστηρίζει ότι στη Σοβιετική Ένωση, αυτοί που προώθησαν αυτές τις προσεγγίσεις καπηλεύτηκαν τη σοσιαλιστική σκέψη ως πηγή έμπνευσης και δικαιολόγησης, ή τουλάχιστον, ως μια βολική πολιτική ασπίδα.

What happened to psychotherapy behind the so-called Iron Curtain? Some commentators have assumed that it was almost non-existent in the Soviet sphere, only to emerge as a significant force in society after the fall of the Berlin Wall (Rose, 1991). Others have written of the vanishing of the unconscious in Eastern Europe, after Freud's work was officially banned by the Communist authorities (Segal, 1975; Wortis, 1953). More recently, these generalisations have been questioned by historians who have begun to mine archives, and conduct interviews with clinicians from the 'psy' professions who practised during the Communist period (Dufaud, 2011; Eghigian, 2002; Eghigian, Killan, & Leuenberger, 2007; Marks & Savelli, 2015; Zajicek, 2009, 2014). This research has unveiled a miscellany of therapeutic approaches, some of which sought to build on socialist philosophies of mind and human nature, and others which positively eschewed Marxism altogether. In this article, I will trace what these contributions, along with primary sources, can tell us about the state of psychotherapy in Communist Europe, and how it survived both underground and above the surface. In particular, I will elaborate on the psychotherapies that were popular across the different countries and language cultures of the Soviet sphere, with a focus upon the Cold War period. This article examines the literature on the mixed fortunes of psychoanalysis and group therapies. More specifically, it reconstructs therapeutic approaches such as suggestion, rational therapy and work therapy, which, in some part, looked to socialist thought as a source of inspiration or, at the very least, as a convenient political shield. Drawing from approaches in the Sociology of Scientific Knowledge (Bloor, 1976/1991), this article does not seek to make normative claims about the psychotherapeutic techniques described, nor does it take a stance in relation to the ethics or politics of the Soviet Union and its satellite countries. Instead, its focuses on exploring the way in which particular modes of treatment survived, or in some cases became ascendant, and the types of justification that were used to support them in the historical context of Communist Europe.

Psychoanalysis: Underground and in plain sight

The sometimes paradoxical fate of psychoanalysis under Communism has been a source of particular fascination for historians and practitioners alike. In the Soviet Union, the initial years after the Bolshevik Revolution saw a surprising level of tolerance and state-sponsored experimentation with Freudian concepts. Accusations of idealism were levelled by Marxist–Leninist philosophers in the critical literature in the 1920s, but for a number of years after 1917, theories of the unconscious and childhood sexuality were not, in fact, seen to be extraneous to the revolutionary project (Etkind, 1997; Launer, 2015; Miller, 1998; Proctor, 2016). The most striking case study is the Children's House (*Detski Dom*) experiment in Moscow, a therapeutic residential institution for children led by the psychoanalytic educationalist Vera Schmidt. With many attendees from among the children of the Party elite, including Stalin's own son, the Children's House pioneered psychoanalytic child rearing practices with involvement from Sabina Spielrein and Alexander Luria (Miller, 1998; Schmidt, 1924; Valkanova, 2016). The project was short-lived, however, with Stalin opting to close it as a demonstration of opposition against Trotsky's vocal support for psychoanalysis. The existence of the Children's House should be considered within the broader context of post-revolutionary debates about the reform of the family, communal living and the collective responsibility for child rearing (Miller, 1998). (And it also, later, provided a source of inspiration for Wilhelm Reich and radical student movements in 1968) (Valkanova, 2016).

Stalin's ascent to power after the death of Lenin in 1924 saw a radical revision of policy, with psychoanalysis officially blacklisted, and Pavlovian techniques elevated in status as the politically acceptable form of approach in the clinical 'psy' disciplines by the 1950s (Zajicek, 2009). In the countries of Central and Eastern Europe, which came under Communist control in the late 1940s, a number of psychoanalytic circles, and even officially recognised local branches of the International Psychoanalytical Association, had coalesced by the time of the outbreak of war in 1939. Their growth was in part facilitated by their geographical proximity to Vienna, the birthplace and the main geographical locus of psychoanalysis throughout the inter-war period. These communities suffered significant losses during the war, with many of their number losing their lives in the Nazi concentration camps. Others went into exile in the West, with a cohort going on to become key players in building the psychoanalytic movement in the US (Erös, 2016). But some did survive, and remain, in the new People's Democracies of the region, and continued to train and practice in unofficial settings, often behind the closed doors of the asylum, or in individuals' private homes (Kovai, 2015; Leuenberger, 2001; Marks, 2015; Savelli, 2013).

Psychoanalysis also continued to inform practice within institutions, sometimes because mental health was considered sufficiently low down on the political priority list that clinicians were allowed to continue their work unnoticed by the authorities, as in the case of Hungary (Kovai, 2015). In East Germany, many made a deliberate choice to reframe their psychoanalytic practice in different terminology, masking research and practice which was otherwise conceptually unchanged (Leuenberger, 2001). In Czechoslovakia, there was a dramatic innovation and expansion of psychoanalytically informed therapies with state funding, through a nationally supported psychedelic psychiatry project which ran from the mid 1950s through to 1974, primarily using LSD to induce abreaction and accelerate the therapeutic process (Crockford, 2007; Marks, 2015). The material presented by patients in these sessions, sometimes mediated through art therapy, was often interpreted as a manifestation of childhood trauma, but also through frameworks informed by Otto Rank's writings on perinatal experience and birth trauma, the Jungian collective unconscious or even the phylogenetic unconscious reverting back to previous evolutionary states, drawing from Carl Jung and Sándor Ferenczi. These approaches had a striking legacy in the international development of transpersonal psychotherapies, with one of the key proponents, Stanislav Grof, emigrating to the USA in 1967 and continuing his work there, largely shaped by the experiences of the Prague-based projects (Marks, 2015).

In Yugoslavia, a Communist country that remained independent of the Soviet sphere of control, psychoanalysis had unexpected fortunes within state-run facilities (Savelli, 2013). Historian Ana Antic has also argued that analytic concepts came to play a particular role in rehabilitation programmes. There was a congruence, she argues, between the goals of both psychoanalysis and the Yugoslav self-management style of socialism, in terms of reforming individuals by prompting them to re-script their life stories according to a template. In the case of Tito's prison camps at Goli Otok, where psychologists informed the re-education programmes, these techniques crossed the line from therapy to coercion (Antic, 2016a, 2016b).

Work therapies

Work therapy, as one might imagine, came to have special place in Marxist–Leninist oriented societies, with the emphasis they placed upon work as central to healthy human functioning, and the importance of the contribution of the individual to the social collective. That said, the role of Communism in facilitating its emergence as a therapeutic modality in Russia and Eastern Europe should not be overestimated. In many countries, work therapies had already become a routine feature of life in asylums and sanatoria the region, as in much of the rest of Europe, from the nineteenth century. 'Moral Treatment', invented at the York Retreat in the 1790s, gradually grew in popularity elsewhere, often in the form of agricultural therapies carried out in the grounds of institutions. In the lands of Germany and the Habsburg Empire, these approaches to treatment were explicitly incorporated into the design of a number of psychiatric institutions – sometimes designed by prestigious modern architects – by the *fin de siècle* (Engstrom, 2011; Topp, 2011, 2017).

In Russia, too, work therapy predated the 1917 Revolution. During the Soviet period, there were a number of schemes for the employment of psychiatric patients in agricultural colonies and in turbine factories built within the grounds of asylums, where payment in return for labour was a possibility, and patients could join trade unions (Sirotkina & Kokorina, 2015). While work therapy was not an invention of the Communist state, as Irina Sirotkina and Marina Kokorina have shown, it nevertheless withered away with the collapse of the Soviet Union

(2015). While there were contingent reasons for its disappearance, the lack of a collective will to lobby for its continuation is also telling of a move away from institutionalised work therapy internationally by the end of the twentieth century. It also signalled the shift in the ideological landscape of Russia itself. There was no longer any significant investment in the idea that employment should guaranteed by the state. Nor in the belief that labour was fundamental to the positive shaping of the individual's personality, ultimately enabling society to function as a whole.

The group and the collective

Work therapies may have been the obvious candidate to focus on in the search for a 'socialist' psychotherapy. But there are others, too, which have been isolated for examination by historians on the supposition that they may have a particularly political character: most especially group therapies. The primacy of collectivism, somewhat predictably, came to be invoked as a way of justifying and promoting these approaches at times. But we need to be careful not to retrospectively overemphasise the significance of groups, as they by no means came to replace – or even to surpass – individual psychotherapies formed around the patient–practitioner dyad. For Miassischev, one of the key ideologues of Soviet psychotherapy, group approaches were useful primarily as a means of reinforcing the effects of treatments that had already been carried out on an individual basis. Cases could be discussed, and patients with similar pathologies could mutually support each other in group-based sessions, in such a way as to 'normalise social relations' (Misassischev, 1960, p. 19, 20). However, Miassischev stopped short of asserting that the collective nature of the group might itself have therapeutic agency, or even that it could be important as a way of simulating socialist society on a smaller scale. He even added a caveat, a warning that group therapy was flawed because of its 'dependence on Freud' (p. 20).

By contrast, in East Germany, group psychotherapeutic practice was indeed framed more explicitly as being in tune with the goals of socialism, with innovations emerging as a consequence of these imperatives. Christine Leuenberger has charted the development of Intentional Dynamic Group Psychotherapy by Kurt Höck at the Berlin psychotherapeutic unit in the 1970s, not long after it was threatened with closure due to the time and expense taken up by the provision of individual approaches (Geyer, 2011; Leuenberger, 2001, p. 265). The group 'dynamic' was exploited as a therapeutic force in itself: while the therapist guided the patients towards an 'intended' goal, they themselves were merely a facilitator. Placing the focus on the interpersonal, socio-psychological processes which played out within this collective setting, individuals were, in Leuenberger's words, 'retrained to act meaningfully in society ... and generally strengthened so they could partake in industrial production' (p. 265).

Such justifications for the ideological validity of therapies were indeed appealing to clinics and medical schools, who were very much aware of being under the watchful eye of the state. Yet, as Mat Savelli argues for the Yugoslav case, many of the clinicians who established group therapy techniques were motivated by an allegiance to social psychiatry as an approach, rather than socialism as such. Inspiration was often drawn from international sources, including the UK-based analyst S.H. Foulkes, with some therapists having also spent time at the Tavistock Clinic in London (Savelli, in press). The striking popularity of Jacob Moreno's 'psychodrama' across the East European region also testifies to an open-mindedness towards the provenance of techniques. This theatre-based approach, which encouraged individuals to literally act out, and then reflect upon, their emotional conflicts in relation to other group participants, was developed primarily in the United States (Aleksandrowicz, 2009; Kratochvíl, 1977; Lauterbach, 1984; Moreno, 2014). Sources from Czechoslovakia in the later years of socialism also show that an eclectic range of authors from both East and West were familiar. Here, Wilfred Bion and Carl Rogers were just as likely to appear in reference lists as key Soviet authors such as Miassischev, Rozhnov or Makarenko (Kratochvíl, 1977). All of these authors, regardless of origin, were taken seriously as sources of inspiration. Group approaches certainly had their place in the psychotherapeutic armament in the Communist East – much as in the West – but, perhaps somewhat surprisingly, they were rarely theorised in terms of Marxist collectivism.

Suggestion

> The dry and pedantic utterances of a tired physician will not cure a single patient. But suggestions – disturbing, arousing, inspiring suggestions – represent a complex and dynamic system of words and meanings, imagery and motions, as well as a functionally psychological and, consequently, physiological totality capable of combining a dynamic form and a significant content. (Misassischev, 1960)

Suggestion, in various forms, was probably the most widely practiced form of psychotherapy in the Soviet sphere of influence (Aleksandrowicz, 2009; Geyer, 2011; Kondáš, 1997; Winn, 1960). Imported to Russia in the early twentieth century by physicians who had made the pilgrimage to prestigious medical institutions in France and Germany for training, suggestion in waking states, as well as through hypnosis, enchanted both clinical and popular audiences in the 1900s (Sirotkina, 2001, p. 102).

Conditioned reflexes also became a central focus of research of some of the most celebrated scientists in the Soviet Union: Vladimir Bekhterev, Ivan Pavlov and Konstantin Bykov. By 1951, the work of Pavlov and his associates were the only officially sanctioned conceptual basis for medicine and the psy-disciplines in the Soviet Union, rendering suggestion-based therapies the most secure approach to work with in political and economic terms (Zajicek, 2009). A canonical text, Konstantin Platonov's *The Word as a Physiological and Therapeutic Factor: The Theory and Practice of Psychotherapy According to I.P. Pavlov*, was published in Russian in 1957, and translated into English by the Moscow Foreign Languages Publishing House in 1959 (Platonov, 1959). Drawing from a wealth of experimentation carried out in the Soviet Union, Platonov made the case for the fundamental role of a particular form of talking therapy. Pavlov had shown, he argued, that humans shared the same type of higher nervous activity as the rest of the animal kingdom. Man, however, had 'a special socially conditioned addition which shows a qualitative peculiarity. This addition is connected with labour and social activity, concerns the speech function and introduces a new principle into the activity of the cerebral hemispheres' (p. 16).

Laboratory research, according to Platonov, had shown that the utterance of words was 'far from immaterial to the human organism', and could have profound effects on physiology (p. 17). Investigations had, for example, demonstrated that it was the very meaning of the word, rather than its sound, which produced an effect upon the body (Shvarts, 1948, 1949). For example, when a person's skin was pricked by a pin, there was an effect on their blood pressure – a similar, if slightly less marked effect could be generated in response to the utterance of the *word* 'pinprick' (Platonov, 1959, p. 21). While these effects were complex, Platonov and others suggested it was feasible to extrapolate from these findings. Words, they argued, had been shown to have myriad effects on both brain and body, and suggestion could therefore be harnessed for medical purposes. Furthermore, it had the potential to treat all organs of the body, in addition to the neurotic disorders more traditionally associated with psychotherapy (Platonov, 1959; Rozhnov, 1954). While the word 'psychotherapy' was retained, these practices went far beyond the treatment of the psyche alone, becoming applied to a range of somatic ailments.

In East Germany, at the university polyclinic in Jena, similar 'autogenic relaxation' techniques were also pioneered by two internal medicine specialists, Gerhard Klumbies and Helmuth Kleinsorge, who had taken over the psychotherapeutic clinic after the war due to staff shortages. Instead of looking back to Russian and French research, they drew upon the work of Jena's own Johannes Schultz and local German psychosomatic traditions from the pre-war period. The clinic became a centre for both experimentation and training: it hosted workshops for the instruction of physicians and therapists from across the Eastern bloc countries, and some from the West (Geyer, 2011; Kleinsorge & Klumbies, 1962). The Jena clinic also produced vinyl records for the purposes of training individuals in self-hypnosis, with booklets demonstrating positions and breathing exercises (Kleinsorge & Klumbies, 1962). Here, we see how psychotherapy left the clinic in the socialist world, forming the basis of prophylactic practices that could be disseminated widely, and carried out in private. This focus on suggestion for prevention and the positive reinforcement of desired behaviours was a key aspect of psychotherapy under socialism. As an example of the utopian uses of psychotherapy, Aleksandra Brokman has shown how autosuggestion came to be used to train Soviet athletes, illustrating the imperative to use these techniques to shape thoughts and emotions in the interests of 'self perfection', far beyond the context of the hospital and clinic (Brokman, 2017).

Persuasion and rationality

In 1960, the Russian psychotherapist Miassischev claimed that there were two main approaches to therapy in the Soviet world: 'suggestion and persuasion. They differ mainly in the purpose of the activating words. Sometimes they are contrasted as the irrational and the rational' (Misassischev, 1960). The latter – usually described simply as 'rational therapy' – was based, in Pavlovian terms, on the most sophisticated functions of the 'secondary signalling system', the parts of the higher nervous system that were specific to the human species. Through active engagement with these conscious, critical faculties based on the capacity for language, it was believed that patients could be literally persuaded back into sound reasoning, and better mental and physical health. While it was developed most enthusiastically in Soviet Russia, rational therapy was taken up in clinics across the region, especially in Poland and Czechoslovakia (Aleksandrowicz, 2009; Kondáš, 1997).

As was the case for work therapies and suggestion, rational therapy was by no means a Soviet – or even a Russian – invention. It was originally the creation of Paul Dubois, a Swiss medical doctor who practiced in Berne in the early twentieth century. Dubois' method was formulated in direct opposition to suggestion, on ethical grounds, arguing that it gave too much power to the therapist at the expense of the patient's own agency (Dubois, 1908; Müller, 2001; Shamdasani, 2005, p. 10). By strengthening the individual's innate ability for logical reasoning, Dubois argued, they could regain not only a sense of healthy functioning, but also a restoration of their personal autonomy.

Whilst largely forgotten in the West, in the early years of the twentieth century, rational therapy was a worthy competitor to psychoanalysis in terms of its popularity in Europe, and this extended as far Russia. There, its status did not, in fact, diminish to the extent that it had elsewhere by the mid-century (Sirotkina, 2001). Rational therapy, like suggestion, was another technique whose long-term fortunes in the Soviet sphere were considerably more favourable than in its own region of origin. In part, one could account for this as the result of the demise of psychoanalysis as an officially sanctioned approach in the USSR after the mid-1920s (Angelini, 2008). Without such a vociferous and institutionally robust rival in Russia, other psychotherapeutics had more space to develop.

But there were also philosophical reasons underlying the enduring regard for rational therapy. The predominant theory of mind in the Soviet Union, beyond Pavlovian studies of higher nervous activity, was Lenin's 'theory of reflection'.

First elaborated in his book *Materialism and Empirio-Criticism*, Lenin asserted that the mind was able to form a reflection of independent, external world. The accuracy of this reflection was bolstered by the findings of science and logical deduction, but it could never be a flawless, unmediated representation of reality, always remaining an ongoing, dialectical process of best approximations. Nevertheless, without ever attaining a fully exact knowledge of the surrounding world, human beings, according to Lenin, had the capacity to achieve a reliable, working reflection of it (Lenin, 1909).

This conception placed a high value on the capacity for scientific reasoning as an essential feature of what it meant to be human: empirical rationality was fundamental to the Soviet model of the healthy mind. Theoreticians of psychotherapy in the Communist period skilfully appropriated the theory of reflection to explain the underlying processes at play in rational therapy. Mental illness was construed as a the consequence of a fault having occurred in the internal reflection of external reality: through a careful process of demonstrating to the patient how these thoughts or assumptions were not, in fact, supported by empirical evidence, the patient could be fundamentally reasoned out of their neurosis (Lauterbach, 1984).

There are some remarkable similarities between the practice of rational therapy in the East, and Albert Ellis's Rational Emotive Behaviour Therapy, or indeed the closely related Cognitive Therapy techniques, developed in the United States from the 1960s, despite knowledge exchange not having occurred across East and West on these particular matters (Beck, 1979; Ellis, 1971). More specifically, REBT's deference to Stoic philosophy, especially Epictetus' epithet that 'men are not disturbed by things, but the views which they take of them', was explicitly mirrored in Soviet rational therapy debates (Dryden & Still, 2012; Lauterbach, 1984). Ellis also, notably, took retrospective inspiration from Dubois to further develop his techniques, indicating that the latter's work has had more of a legacy than historians have acknowledged (Dryden & Still, 2012). That psychotherapeutic techniques should have come to develop in parallel with each other to such an extent, across the so-called Iron Curtain, may appear counterintuitive. But it can be read as testament to the similar imperatives on both sides for the creation of self-controlled persons, guided by enlightenment ideals of rationality, at the very height of Cold War modernity (see Krylova, 2014).

Conclusions

The fall of the Berlin Wall and the Collapse of the Soviet Union shifted the terrain for the role of psychotherapy in the region. In some post-socialist countries, psychotherapeutic concepts have come to play a new type of function in social life, becoming taken up as a way of trying to work through, and come to terms with, difficult aspects of the Communist past – at both a personal and a national, collective level (Leuenberger, 2000; Marks, 2017). It has also certainly been the case that the collapse of Communism enabled an expansion of psychotherapeutic practice, both in terms of the quantity of professionals offering therapy, and the variety of approaches available in private practice (Rose, 1991). But this isn't, of course, to say that the psychotherapeutic professions, and the knowledge they produced, were absent, or did not hold a stake in society under socialism (Buda, Tomcsanyi, Harmatta, Csaky-Pallavicini, & Paneth, 2009; Calloway, 1993; Doboş, 2015; Raikhel & Bemme, 2016).

Adéla Gjuričová, writing on the last two decades of the Communist regime in Czechoslovakia, reminds us that some forms of therapy existed with norms of private payment for years before the emergence of an official free market economy, suggesting that these forms of transaction might have paved the way for the acceptance and proliferation of private practice in the 1990s (Gjuričová, in press). As noted above, a plurality of techniques – including some that the state was officially hostile towards – existed both underground and semi-officially in most countries, even if those practising them were only afforded limited degrees of freedom. But there are other distinctive continuities between the socialist and post-socialist periods. The clear resonances between Pavlovian and suggestion-based therapies with behavioural approaches, as well as between rational therapies and cognitive approaches, meant that clinicians trained in these techniques were able to rebrand themselves as cognitive and behavioural therapists in the 1990s, with some even framing the former as 'predecessors' to the latter in their own histories of the profession (Kondáš, 1997).

It is also important not to underplay the continuities and similarities in practice across East and West, in some cases facilitated by exchange of knowledge and personnel across borders. In other instances, this was more a legacy of pre-Communist, trans-European intellectual networks, especially engagement with French and German language cultures, dating back to the late nineteenth and early twentieth centuries. And yet, for certain approaches, particularly those based on suggestion, rational persuasion, or the value of work, the socialist context – and the philosophies fostered by the Soviet Union and its satellites – did tangibly shape the development of therapeutic theory and practice. For all of the limitations and restrictions places on intellectual freedom within the Soviet sphere, in these cases, socialism was itself a muse for innovation.

Disclosure statement

No potential conflict of interest was reported by the author.

Funding

This work was supported by the Wellcome Trust [grant number 103344/Z/13/Z].

References

Aleksandrowicz, J. W. (2009). The history of polish psychotherapy during the socialist dictatorship. *European Journal of Mental Health, 4*(1), 57–66.

Angelini, A. (2008). History of the unconscious in Soviet Russia: From its origins to the fall of the Soviet Union. *International Journal of Psychoanalysis, 89*(2), 369–388.

Antic, A. (2016a). The pedagogy of workers' self-management: Terror, therapy, and reform communism in Yugoslavia after the Tito-Stalin split. *Journal of Social History, 50*, 179–203.

Antic, A. (2016b). Therapeutic violence: Psychoanalysis and the 're-education' of political prisoners in cold war Yugoslavia and Eastern Europe. In M. ffytche & D. Pick (Eds.), *Psychoanalysis in the age of totalitarianism* (pp. 163–178) Abingdon: Routledge.

Beck, A. T. (1979). *Cognitive therapy of depression*. New York, NY: Guilford Press.

Bloor, D. (1976/1991). *Knowledge and social imagery* (2nd ed.). Chicago, IL: University of Chicago Press.

Brokman, A. (2017). Psychotherapy for champions: suggestion and self-perfection in the training of soviet athletes. *Hidden Persuaders Blog*. http://www.bbk.ac.uk/hiddenpersuaders/blog/psychotherapy-champions-autosuggestion-self-perfection-training-soviet-athletes/

Buda, B., Tomcsanyi, T., Harmatta, J., Csaky-Pallavicini, R., & Paneth, G. (2009). Psychotherapy in hungary during the socialist era and the socialist dictatorship. *European Journal of Mental Health, 4*(1), 67–99.

Calloway, P. (1993). *Russian/Soviet and western psychiatry: A contemporary comparative study*. London: Wiley.

Crockford, R. (2007). LSD in Prague: A long-term follow-up study. *Multidisciplinary Association for Psychedelic Studies, 12*(1), 20–22.

Doboş, C. (2015). Psychiatry and ideology: The emergence of 'Asthenic Neurosis' in communist Romania. In M. Savelli & S. Marks (Eds.), *Psychiatry in communist Europe* (pp. 93–116). Basingstoke: Palgrave.

Dryden, W., & Still, A. (2012). *The historical and philosophical context of rational psychotherapy: The legacy of Epictetus*. London: Karnac.

Dubois, P. (1908). *The psychiatric treatment of nervous disorders*. New York, NY, NY: Funk & Wagnells.

Dufaud, G. (2011). "Un retour aux anciennes maisons de fous"? Réformer les institutions psychiatriques en Russie soviétique (1918–1928). *Revue historique, 4*, 875–897. doi:10.3917/rhis.114.0875

Eghigian, G. (2002). Was there a communist psychiatry? Politics and east German psychiatric care, 1945–1989. *Harvard Review of Psychiatry, 10*, 364–368.

Eghigian, G., Killan, A., & Leuenberger, C. (2007). The self as project: Politics and the human sciences in the twentieth century. *Osiris, 22*, 1–25.

Ellis, A. (1971). *Growth through Reason: Verbatim cases in rational-emotive therapy*. Palo Alto: Science and Behaviour Books.

Engstrom, E. (2011). Placing psychiatric practice: On the spatial configurations and contests of professional labour in late-nineteenth century Germany. In L. Topp, J. E. Moran, & J. Andrews (Eds.), *Madness, architecture and the built environment: Psychiatric spaces in historical context* (pp. 63–82). Abingdon: Routledge.

Erös, F. (2016). Psychoanalysis and the emigration of central and eastern European intellectuals. *The American Journal of Psychoanalysis, 76*(4), 399–413.

Etkind, A. (1997). *Eros of the impossible: History of psychoanalysis in Russia*. Boulder, CO: Westview.

Geyer, M. (Ed.). (2011). *Psychotherapie in Ostdeutschland*. Kornwestheim: Vandenhoeck & Ruprecht.

Gjuričová, A. (in press). Bohatství pod neviditelným pláštěm? Psychoterapie v Československu po roce 1968. *Časopis pro soudobé dějiny*.

Kleinsorge, H., & Klumbies, G. (1962). *Technik der Relaxation: Selbstentspannung*. Jena: Fischer.

Kondáš, O. (1997). Cognitive and behaviour therapy in Slovakia: A historical overview. *Studia Psychologica, 39*, 247–256.

Kovai, M. (2015). The history of the Hungarian institute of psychiatry and neurology between 1945 and 1968. In M. Savelli & S. Marks (Eds.), *Psychiatry in communist Europe* (pp. 117–133). Basingstoke: Palgrave.

Kratochvíl, S. (1977). *Skupinová psychoterapie neuros*. Prague: Avicenum.

Krylova, A. (2014). Soviet modernity: Stephen Kotkin and the Bolshevik predicament. *Contemporary European History, 23*, 167–192.

Launer, J. (2015). *Sex versus survival: The life and ideas of Sabina Spielrein*. London: Overlook.

Lauterbach, W. (1984). *Soviet psychotherapy*. Oxford: Pergamon.

Lenin, V. I. (1909). *Materialism and empirio-criticsim: Critical comments on a reactionary philosophy*.

Leuenberger, C. (2000). The Berlin wall on the therapist's couch. *Human Studies, 23*, 99–121.

Leuenberger, C. (2001). Socialist psychotherapy and its dissidents. *Journal of the History of the Behavioural Sciences, 37*, 267–373. doi:10.1002/jhbs.1034

Marks, S. (2015). From experimental psychosis to resolving traumatic pasts: Psychedelic research in communist Czechoslovakia, 1954–1974. *Cahiers du monde russe, 53*–75.

Marks, S. (2017). The Romani minority, coercive sterilization, and languages of denial in the Czech lands. *History Workshop Journal, 84*, 128–148.

Marks, S., & Savelli, M. (2015). Communist Europe and transnational psychiatry. In M. Savelli & S. Marks (Eds.), *Psychiatry in communist Europe* (pp. 1–26). Basingstoke: Palgrave.

Miller, M. (1998). *Freud and the Bolsheviks: Psychoanalysis in imperial Russia and the Soviet Union*. New Haven, CT: Yale University Press.

Misassischev in Winn, R., (Ed.). (1960). *Psychotherapy in the Soviet Union*. London: Peter Owen.

Moreno, J. D. (2014). *Impromptu man: J. L. Moreno and the origins of psychodrama, encounter culture, and the social network*. New York, NY: Belleview Literary Press.

Müller, C. (2001). *"Sie müssen an Ihre Heilung glauben!": Paul Dubois; ein vergessener Pionier der Psychotherapie*. Basel: Schwabe.

Platonov, K. (1959). *The word as a physiological and therapeutic factor: The theory and practice of psychotherapy according to I.P. Pavlov*. Moscow: Foreign Languages Publishing House.

Proctor, H. (2016). 'A country beyond the pleasure principle': Alexander Luria, death drive and dialectic in Soviet Russia, 1917–1930. *Psychoanalysis and History, 18*, 155–182. doi:10.3366/pah.2016.0187

Raikhel, E., & Bemme, D. (2016). Postsocialism, the psy-ences and mental health. *Transcultural Psychiatry, 53*, 151–175. doi:10.1177/1363461516635534

Rose, N. (1991). Experts of the soul. *Psychologie und Geschichte, 3*(1/2), 91–99.

Rozhnov, V. E. (1954). *Gipnoz v meditsine*. Moscow: Medgiz.

Savelli, M. (2013). The peculiar prosperity of psychoanalysis in socialist Yugoslavia. *The Slavonic and East European Review, 91*, 262–288. doi:10.5699/slaveasteurorev2.91.2.0262

Savelli, M. (in press). "Peace and happiness await us somewhere in the distant future and at that level psychotherapy can act": Psychotherapy in Yugoslavia, 1945–1985. *History of the Human Sciences*.

Schmidt, V. (1924). *Psychoanalytical education in Soviet Russia*. London: International Psychoanalytic Press.

Segal, B. M. (1975). The theoretical basis of soviet psychotherapy. *American Journal of Psychotherapy, 29*(4), 503–523.

Shamdasani, S. (2005). Psychotherapy: The invention of a word. *History of the Human Sciences, 18*(1), 1–22. doi:10.1177/0952695105051123

Shvarts, A. A. (1948). Znachenie slova I ego zvukovo obraza kak uslovnovo razdrazhitelya. *Byulleten eksperimentalnoi biologii i meditsini, 4*

Shvarts, A. A. (1949). Smisl slova I ego zvukovoi obraza kak uslovnie razdrzhiteli, Soobshenie 2, *Byulleten eksperimentalnoi biologii i meditsini, 6*.

Sirotkina, I. (2001). *Diagnosing literary genius: A cultural history of psychiatry in Russia, 1880–1930*. Baltimore, MD: Johns Hopkins University Press.

Sirotkina, I., & Kokorina, M. (2015). The dialectics of labour in a psychiatric ward: Work therapy in the Kashchenko hospital. In M. Savelli & S. Marks (Eds.). *Psychiatry in communist Europe* (pp. 27–49). Basingstoke: Palgrave.

Topp, L. (2011). The modern mental hospital in late-nineteenth century Germany and Austria: Psychiatric space and images of freedom and control. In L. Topp, J. E. Moran, & J. Andrews (Eds.), *Madness, architecture and the built environment: Psychiatric spaces in historical context* (pp. 241–262). Abingdon: Routledge.

Topp, L. (2017). *Freedom and the cage: Modern architecture and psychiatry in central Europe, 1890–1914*. Philadelphia, PA: Penn State University Press.

Valkanova, Y. (2016). The psychoanalytic kindergarten project in Soviet Russia 1921–1930. *SCRSS Digest, 2*, 12–15.

Winn, R. (Ed.). (1960). *Psychotherapy in the Soviet Union*. London: Peter Owen.

Wortis, J. (1953). *Soviet psychiatry*. Baltimore, MD: Williams & Wilkins.

Zajicek, B. (2009). *Scientific psychiatry in Stalin's Soviet Union: The politics of modern medicine and the struggle to define "Pavlovian" psychiatry, 1939–1953*. (PhD Thesis). University of Chicago.

Zajicek, B. (2014). Soviet madness: Nervousness, mild schizophrenia, and the professional jurisdiction of psychiatry in the USSR, 1918–1936. *Ab Imperio, 2014*, 167–194.

Manualizing psychotherapy: Aaron T. Beck and the origins of *Cognitive Therapy of Depression*

Rachael I. Rosner

ABSTRACT

This paper examines the origins of psychiatrist Aaron T. Beck's 1979 Cognitive Therapy of Depression (CTOD). CTOD was the first psychotherapy manual designed to be used in a randomized controlled trial (RCT). Making psychotherapy amenable to the RCT design had been a 'holy grail' for leading American psychotherapy researchers since the late 1960s. Beck's CTOD – which standardized his treatment so it could be compared with drug treatments in a clinical trial – delivered that holy grail, and ushered in the manualized treatment revolution. Manuals are now a sine qua non in psychotherapy research. In this paper, I explore some of the personal, political, and economic variables that made the idea of a manual irresistible to Beck and to those who first championed him.

LA MANUALIZACION DE LA PSICOTERAPIA

En este artículo se examinan los orígenes del libro TERAPIA COGNITIVA DE LA DEPRESION (TCD)del psiquiatra americano Aaron T. Beck (1979). Este libro fue el primer manual de psicoterapia a ser utilizado en un experimento controlado al azar (ECA). Desde los años sesenta, destacados investigadores americanos en psicoterapia, habían estado tratando de encontrar "el cáliz sagrado" que podría hacer la psicoterapia malleable para los ECA. El libro de Beck (TCD), el cual estandarizaba los tratamientos para poder ocmpararlos con los de drogas en un ECA, parecía haber encontrado ese "cáliz sagrado" y de esta manera inició la revolución del tratamiento según un manual. Los manuales son actualmente un 'sine qua non' en la investigación en psicoterapia. En este artículo se exploran algunas de las variables personales, políticas y económicas que hicieron que la idea de un manual fuese irresistible para Beck y aquéllos que le dieron su apoyo desde los comienzos.

La psicoterapia manualizzata: Aaron T. Beck e le origini della Terapia Cognitiva della Depressione

Questo articolo esamina le origini della Terapia Cognitiva della Depressione (CTOD) proposta dallo psichiatra Aaron T. Beck nel 1979. CTOD è stato il primo manuale di psicoterapia progettato per essere utilizzato in uno studio randomizzato controllato (RCT). Rendere la psicoterapia soggetta a disegni di ricerca RCT è stato un "sacro graal" per la ricerca americana sulla psicoterapia sin dalla fine degli anni '60. Il CTOD di Beck, che standardizzava il suo trattamento in modo che potesse essere paragonato ai trattamenti farmacologici sottoposti a in una sperimentazione clinica, con quel santo graal inaugurava una rivoluzione relativa ai manuali di trattamento. I manuali sono ora una condizione *sine qua non* nella ricerca in psicoterapia. In questo articolo esploro alcune delle variabili personali, politiche ed economiche che hanno reso la predisposizione di un manuale un'idea irrinunciabile per Beck e per coloro che per primi lo hanno sostenuto.

Manualiser la thérapie: Aaron T. Beck et les origines de la thérapie cognitive pour la dépression

Cet article examine les origines de la Thérapie Cognitive pour la Dépression (CTOD) du psychiatre Aaron T. Beck en 1979. CTOD est le premier manuel psychothérapeutique qui fut élaboré afin d'être utilisé dans les essais randomisés contrôlés (RCT). Rendre la psychothérapie compatible avec les paramètres des RCT constituait le « Saint Graal » pour les chercheurs en psychothérapie américains de renom depuis la fin des années 60. La CTOD de Beck - qui standardisait son traitement afin qu'il soit comparable aux traitements médicamenteux lors d'un essai clinique - fournît ce Saint Graal et introduisit la révolution du traitement manualisé. Les manuels sont à présent un sine qua non de la recherche en psychothérapie. Dans cet article, j'explore quelques-unes des variables personnelles, politiques et économiques qui rendirent l'idée d'un manuel irrésistible pour Beck et pour ceux qui le soutinrent dans ses débuts.

Ψυχοθεραπεία: AaronBeckκαι οι απαρχές της Γνωστικής Θεραπείας της Κατάθλιψης

ΠΕΡΙΛΗΨΗ
Αυτό το άρθρο εξετάζει την προέλευση της Γνωστικής Θεραπείας της Κατάθλιψης που προτάθηκε από τονAaronT. Beck το 1979. Η Γνωστική Θεραπεία της Κατάθλιψης αποτελεί το πρώτο ψυχοθεραπευτικό εγχειρίδιο που σχεδιάστηκε με σκοπό να χρησιμοποιηθεί σε τυχαιοποιημένη δοκιμή με ομάδα ελέγχου. Η υπαγωγή της ψυχοθεραπείας σε τυχαιοποιημένες δοκιμές με ομάδα ελέγχου αποτέλεσε το «ιερό δισκοπότηρο» που καθοδήγησε τους Αμερικανούς ερευνητές της ψυχοθεραπείας από τα τέλη της δεκαετίας του 1960. Η Γνωστική Θεραπεία της Κατάθλιψης που προτάθηκε από τον Beck - η οποία αποτελεί στανταρισμένη θεραπεία η οποία μπορεί να συγκριθεί με τη φαρμακοθεραπεία σε κλινικές δοκιμές- παρέλαβε αυτό το «ιερό δισκοπότηρο» και οδήγησε στην επανάσταση της ψυχοθεραπείας με βάση εγχειρίδια. Τα πρωτόκολλα αποτελούν τώρα απαραίτητη προϋπόθεση στην έρευνα της ψυχοθεραπείας. Σε αυτό το άρθρο, εξετάζω μερικές από τις προσωπικές, πολιτικές και οικονομικές μεταβλητές που κατέστησαν την ιδέα του πρωτοκόλλου ακαταμάχητη για τον Beck και σε αυτούς που πρώτοι τον υπερασπίστηκαν.

In the early 1970s, leading American psychotherapy researchers and policy-makers began an all-out effort to figure out how to make psychotherapy, one of the most private and subjective experiences, amenable to one of the most public and quantitative scientific methods, the randomized-controlled trial (RCT) (Bergin & Strupp, 1972; Fiske et al., 1970; Rosner, 2005). The question of whether or not it was possible or even advisable to quantify psychotherapy had been on scientists' radar since the mid-1950 (Rosner, 2005). Psychoanalysts, who dominated American psychotherapy at that time, argued that applying experimental processes to psychotherapy would destroy the very thing they were trying to measure, namely the transference relationship between therapist and patient – an argument akin to the Heisenberg principle. Even as late as the mid-1960s, in three NIMH-sponsored conferences on psychotherapy research, researchers couldn't agree on the value of experiments in psychotherapy. Psychoanalytic researchers disavowed them as an assault on subjectivity. Behavior therapists overwhelmingly championed them precisely for the same reason (Rosner, 2005).

The rising influence of the Food and Drug Administration (FDA) in the wake of the thalidomide crisis of the early 1960s, followed by the heat of the Viet Nam War on government coffers, forced these debates to take a backseat to the problem of aligning psychotherapy with new national standards for medical and drug research (Bothwell, Greene, Podolsky, & Jones, 2016; Fiske et al., 1970; Greene & Podolsky, 2012; Marks, 1997). Congress and NIH administrators were demanding accountability and the RCT became the method of choice – even as skepticism about RCTs within the medical community remained (Bothwell et al., 2016; Jones, 2000). Concern over accountability grew even more urgent when President Carter began pushing for national health insurance in 1976. A broad spectrum of medical specialties from asthma to diabetes, psychotherapy among them, was now under intense pressure to adapt to the RCT design[1] (Parloff, 1979; Marks, 1997).

The technology that delivered this holy grail to psychotherapists came out of the laboratory of psychiatrist Aaron T. Beck of the University of Pennsylvania, founder of Cognitive Therapy (CT) and father-figure of the Cognitive-Behavior Therapy (CBT) movement. CT was a new approach to therapy that emphasized brief courses of treatment focused on changing patients' thinking and behavior. In the mid-1970s, Beck created a 'manualized' treatment for the study of his new cognitive therapy of depression (CTOD), such that every patient received the same treatment on the same days of a prescribed course of treatment under randomized conditions. His new manualized approach was tested at the federal level in the first multi-site RCT of psychotherapy. And the published version of his manual, his 400-page CTOD (Beck, Rush, Shaw, & Emery, 1979), became a best seller and the gold standard. Psychotherapy manuals are now so ubiquitous in this era of evidence-based medicine that they function a bit like philosopher Bruno Latour's 'black box' (Latour, 1987), a technology whose usefulness is so self-evident that few pay heed to its mechanics.

In this essay, I venture into the origins of Beck's CTOD. My aim is not to uncover its mechanics, nor to offer a prelude to the heated debates over manuals that continue to this day (Addis, Wade, & Hatgis, 1999; Barlow & Green, 2001; Dobson & Shaw, 1988; Kazdin, 2008; Parloff, 1998; Silverman, 1996; Strupp & Anderson, 1997; Westen & Bradley, 2005; Wilson, 1998), but rather to explore simply why Beck, and those who championed him, found this particular solution to the RCT problem so compelling in the first place. My argument is that CTOD, from the moment of its inception through its publication and beyond, was a potent, public and deliberate snub of the old order: where psychotherapy had emphasized subjectivity and irrationality, Beck would champion objectivity and reason; where psychoanalysts thrived on secrecy and hierarchy, Beck and his followers would demand accountability and democracy; where philosopher-king-therapists concentrated power, they would now distribute power; and where therapists had once eschewed drugs, they would make psychotherapy behave just like drugs (and even exceed their potency). Drugs were now on the upswing in the treatment of mental problems, and both Beck and NIMH policy-makers knew that making psychotherapy behave like drugs could demonstrate its prowess in this new medical climate.

CTOD was the first of what I call *second-generation manuals*. First-generation manuals – the first manuals so designated – emerged in the 1960s among behavior therapists. Behavior therapists were psychologists (not medical doctors, like psychoanalysts) applying the principles of Pavlov, Watson and Skinner to clinical practice. They were among the founders of the Society for Psychotherapy Research (SPR) in 1969. The purpose of their manuals was very specific: to outline the steps of a specific intervention to standardize it for experimental research. The very first manual (Paul, 1966) was part of a study comparing behavioral and psychodynamic interventions for public speaking anxiety. But neither this manual nor those first-generation manuals which succeeded it were designed for clinical trials. Neither did they describe nor delineate the techniques of a therapy in its entirety.[2] They had a more focal purpose. Our story begins in the next phase, the 1970s, when Aaron Beck repurposed the idea of a manual. Revolutionary virtues attended upon his manual that did not inhere in first-generation ones.

Beck's manual for CTOD

Aaron Beck began his career at Penn in the mid-1950s as a psychoanalyst. He specialized in the treatment of depression and conducted psychoanalytic research. As his research progressed, Beck suspected that depression might be a thought disorder – not as severe as schizophrenia but nonetheless evidencing distortions in thought – rather than a mood disorder. Following several professional crises in the early 1960s, he turned his back on organized psychoanalysis. He took a five-year sabbatical (1962–1967) to pursue new ideas about cognitions in depression (Beck, 1967; Rosner, 2012, 2014). He published the two foundational articles on thinking and depression (Beck, 1963, 1964) and his first book (Beck, 1967) during this period of 'splendid isolation'. This was the period in which cognitive therapy was born.

Beck's frustration with psychoanalysis lay in its culture of dogmatism and loyalty. The professional crises he experienced in the early 1960s were the by-product of a postwar psychoanalytic establishment that held too much power and abused that power with apparent abandon (see Hale, 1995)[3]. The analysts in Beck's orbit who sat in positions of power preached that psychoanalytic theory (especially the unconscious) was inviolable, experimental data were viable only if they supported the theory (and should be thrown out, if not), and skepticism and critique were to be curtailed (with strong-arm tactics, if necessary). Secrecy, not accountability, held sway. But for Beck personally, in virtually all respects – in his own personal course of psychoanalytic treatment, in his closest friendship at Penn, in his relationships with psychoanalytic and psychiatric mentors, even in his application for membership in the American Psychoanalytic Association – this same set of virtues was not bringing success but rather harm to himself, to his patients, to his collegial relationships, and to his professional prospects. And so it was the political stranglehold on innovation, science, skeptical inquiry, and self-determination that ultimately led Beck to turn his back on organized psychoanalysis (Rosner, 2014).

So whatever grievances Beck ultimately had with psychoanalysis – theoretical, clinical, and scientific – it was this stranglehold on his own professional advancement that sparked the fire of Beck's new cognitive therapy. From 1962 on, Beck's sole business was to create and promote a new 'enlightened' worldview to govern how therapists should work with patients, with ideas, with scientific data, and with each other. First and foremost, Beck championed empiricism, objectivity and experimentalism. These were the cornerstones that would guarantee accountability. And there would be a distinctly democratic flavor to this experimentalism: to experiment implied to collaborate, to collaborate implied to work openly (and not in secret), and to work openly implied discussion and debate. And quantified data would supplant unanchored theoretical speculation as the basis for clinical judgment (Rosner, 2014). This new set of expectations suffused Beck's two articles (1963, 1964) and his first book (1967), and are the backdrop for understanding the power behind CTOD.

When Beck returned to academic life in 1967 following his five-year sabbatical, he had high expectations that cognitive therapy would find a warm reception. Philadelphia in the late 1960s was a fertile breeding ground of psychotherapies, as well as a hotbed of experimental psychotherapy research. Under the chairmanship of Albert J. (Mickey) Stunkard, Penn's psychiatry department hosted an eclectic group of psychotherapy researchers all pushing various corners of experimental science, including Lester Luborsky, Martin Orne, John Paul Brady, and Salvador Minuchin (family therapy). Temple University across town had also recently welcomed Joseph Wolpe, the South African father of behavior therapy, and his compatriot protégé Arnold Lazarus, who later broke with Wolpe to pursue his own school of therapy called Multimodal Therapy.

Political polarities in Philadelphia made such a warm welcome impossible, however. Beck actively courted Wolpe, for instance, but disagreements over theory and practice made headway difficult. Beck brought CT to his local psychoanalytic society, positioning CT as a new variant of psychoanalysis predicated on experimentalism; but, he later recalled, local analysts concluded that CT was no such thing.[4] So, Beck turned to his students. He offered a seminar to 2nd year psychiatry residents in 'Broad Spectrum Psychotherapy', or what students called the 'Systems' course. Beck invited a parade of luminaries (including Albert Ellis of New York City, founder of Rational Emotive Therapy) to do live demonstrations with patients. Of course he included his own cognitive therapy. And his students uniformly liked the course. But the majority remained psychoanalytically-inclined.[5] This was hardly a giant wave of enthusiasm.

The point here is that Beck did not merely germinate a new school of psychotherapy predicated on ideas of democracy and accountability – he also promoted this new approach in a fertile breeding ground and scientific environment with full expectations that someone eventually would follow. He was fomenting a revolution in psychiatry, and he used every method to generate a following. This long list of early failures is actually evidence of how persistently and urgently he sought a following.

Beck's revolutionary party finally got started in Philadelphia in 1973.[6] A second year psychiatry resident named John Rush took Beck's Systems course. Rush grew enamored of CT and was convinced it was more effective than psychoanalysis, drugs or ECT. He and a fellow resident, Manoocheer Khatami, had recently set up a low-fee depression clinic on nights and weekends on Penn's campus. They asked Beck to supervise them in CT:

> (We said) 'what we'll do is open a depression clinic for uninsured blue-collar people.' So what we did is, we pan-handled ourselves around … So we said, 'Alright, we have 4 great people. We have Tim Beck,' who hadn't yet coined the term cognitive therapy, but we knew he was doing weird stuff because the patients were actually sitting up and talking to him, and he's assigning homework. We're watching him through a one-way mirror (and) if they had a panic attack he'd ring the bell to break off the attack. And I'm going 'This doesn't look like psychoanalysis to me, it's not even psychodynamic. I don't know, they should get worse not better.' But his patients were getting better … 'So we gotta get Tim Beck, he knows about depression, and he wrote the book on depression, he's got the depression inventory, we can't move forward without Tim Beck.' He seemed like a nice man with a little red tie and the gray hair.

Rush also urged Beck to undertake an RCT comparing CT with drugs. Rush had just learned the RCT methodology for drug trials from another professor at Penn, yet another South African psychiatrist named Joe Mendels. Rush asked Beck to consider the possibility:

> I said, 'We gotta find out if this really works.' He says, 'What does that mean?' I say, 'You know, like Joe Mendels, a drug trial.' Because I learned about drug trials from Mendels, learning about placebo controls and structured interviewing, and there was a whole new thing called a SADS interview, and that was part of the NIMH collaborative [study of the psychopharmacology of depression], and Joe was part of that … So all of that was cool, and so Tim says, and this is the very important part: "That"s a good idea.' I didn't know how radical that statement was, because he had been working on this (already) for 20 years. I'm just a slightly brazen little bit older, very naive resident who says, 'This is exciting!' I've got three patients that failed ECT, whoa! Plus another one was also tough, now they're really a whole lot better. I said 'Maybe this works.'

There was no money to fund the trial, no research team, no coterie of therapists trained in cognitive therapy – it would be from scratch:

> (I said) are you sure, you gray-haired fool, that this actually works? I am the skep-tic right? And he's saying sure, I'll put the last twenty years of my life on the line, I'm just a scientist. And I thought, you know, there is nobody – nobody – (who) does that today. That is a big risk, especially to turn it over to a nut resident. I am unskilled, I had never done a randomized trial in my life, right? … So then he said – we were kind of talking together, so I can't remember who said what – but we said, 'We have to figure out how to do this with no money. Because there's no grant.' So I think I said, 'The residents love to work with you. You can supervise the residents. I can sweet talk them into the drugs. We'll just randomize it.'

This is the context in which Beck's manual emerged. Having decided to under-take a clinical trial, Beck and Rush needed to standardize CT. So Rush came up with a plan:

> … Early on I said 'We have to write down what you're doing with the residents because nobody can replicate it. Because even if you find something, nobody will care …' It [CT] hadn't been written down. It was all in his head. He would just show up and he would create these things with the patient … So we just decided, I think it was Tim, we'll just keep notes.[7]

On 12 October 1973 Beck crafted his first outline, a modest four page 'Protocol for Cognitive Behavioral Therapy of Depression: Rough draft'.[8] The first page offered his 'rationale' for CT: 'The goal of therapy through the use of activity schedules and cognitive techniques is to undermine the patient's faulty belief system that contributes to his distorted, negative, conceptualizations'. The remaining three pages listed a 'General Resume of Techniques'. A few weeks later Beck generated an expanded 'Protocol for Cognitive-Behavioral Therapy of Depression' which he renamed 'Treatment Manual for Cognitive-Behavioral Therapy of Depression'.[9] Beck mentored Rush in his writing skills and supervised a case study that Rush and Khatami published (Rush et al., 1975). They also collaborated on the manual, which grew in size with every draft. In one version they outlined the steps down to the minute.

The manual turned out to be a potent vehicle for publicizing CT. It was like an invitation to an ongoing party. In 1977, for instance, Beck dispatched students to conferences with 3x5 cards advertising the unpublished manual at $9 per copy. He also advertised the manual in his articles as, for instance, in a footnote in his team's 1977 article announcing the results of their trial (Rush, Beck, Kovacs, & Hollon, 1977).[10] This publicity effectively stirred up interest outside Beck's inner circle. David M. Clark, a British psychologist, remembers:

> Many of the students thought it'd be really nice if we could learn a bit about this [CT], because our professors didn't know it. There was actually a manual available, a mimeographed manual where you could send a check to Barbara Marinelli at the center [for cognitive therapy] and they would send you this mimeographed version … which was straight genius on Tim's behalf. So I got together a group of people and we made out an international money order, which was difficult to do in those days, and I think we ordered ten copies. So we were then the most popular students because we had the gold. And we lent it out and tried to learn it. We read it and tried to use it with patients. It seemed to work quite well with depressed patients, so we were very impressed.[11]

The manual also instantiated a prime directive of CT, namely, collaboration. To imagine that therapy might be a collaborative enterprise with an equal distribution of power between therapist and patient was radical at the time. Beck was working with patients as collaborators in the laboratory of their own lives. There would no longer be secrets but consensus.[12] In collaborating on the manual, Beck's students experienced that same directive – between mentor and mentee as much as therapist and patient – first-hand. Beck extended the collaboration to every resident, post-doctoral fellow, medical student and psychology undergraduate who entered his laboratory. He needed their insights and they gained ownership in the evolution of the model.

Beck invited Maria Kovacs, a recent Ph.D. who Beck had hired to coordinate an ongoing study of drug-addiction and suicide, to join the team, while Rush corralled fellow residents. On 1 August 1974 Rush and Khatami's off-hours low-fee depression clinic became the 'Mood Clinic'.[13] The Mood Clinic's purpose was to treat depressed patients with CT or drugs for this first clinical trial. Rush, Khatami, Kovacs and two other residents were the therapists. Lester Luborsky (the most experienced psychotherapy researcher at Penn) and Karl Rickels (an expert in psychopharmacology) consulted.

Beck's first task was to 'develop a standard "Instruction Manual" for training therapists in cognitive-behavioral (C/B) therapy of depression and anxiety'. Beck wanted to know everything his students observed in clinic, every obstacle, every failure and success with patients. He instructed them to ask their patients directly about whether or not the therapists' formulations made sense. He asked them to forward clinical vignettes to Rush to include in the manual, and to critique its revisions:

The special precepting sessions with Dr. Beck will be sources of instruction, specification of methodologies for the manual and development of new C/B techniques. It is anticipated that the 'Manual' may form the basis of added training for future residents. Dr. Rush will collect notes from the therapists involved … and be responsible for converting the collective clinical experience of the group into the 'Treatment Manual.' Revisions of the treatment manual will be circulated every 3-4 months.[14]

Beck also gathered everyone once a week for a brain-storming session:

> He started to have a weekly meeting (where) he … would talk about the patients that he saw, he would talk about the ideas. I was the person who took notes. Part of how the manual came around is … we would actually try out some of the stuff. Tim would say, 'Go ahead and try this.' And I'd go and I would try this with my patient and then I'd come back and I would say, 'you know what, this really works!' And then everybody would go 'wow!' Or I would say, 'You know what Tim, you really should give this (exercise) a name, like we should call this the Triple Column, or Double Column, this really should have a name.' So we would start coming up with names, and then there were times when he would suggest something, and it didn't work. So that's how actually the manual came about.[15]

In June 1974 the manual was 46 pages. By May 1975 it had grown to 89 pages, just in time for the team to present their preliminary findings, at the annual meeting of SPR in 1975 in Boston, that CT was more effective than drugs with depression.[16]

The manual continued to expand after the original group's departure and after the Mood Clinic was renamed the Center for Cognitive Therapy. Rush left in July 1975. That same year a pre-doctoral psychology student named Steve Hollon and a psychologist named Brian Shaw from Toronto joined. Hollon became clinic coordinator, and one of Shaw's jobs was to write the manual:

> 1976 was the big push to get the manual. And the process was I would write something, I would give it to either Marika or Tim or both of them, they would give feedback … Tim would send a note back or discuss it, or he would role-play. He loved to role-play. And so a lot of our time was spent where – this is actually so precious to me, it's so funny – he would be the depressed person, or I would be a depressed person. Both of us could be excellent depressed people.[17]

Shaw stayed through 1976; Hollon left in 1977. Kovacs left in 1977 and a pre-doctoral psychology student named Gary Emery joined. Emery stayed into the mid-1980s. A medical student named Ira Herman and a resident named David Burns joined, and a wave of clinical psychologists came in including Arthur Freeman (who had been trained and treated by Albert Ellis), Rich Bedrosian, and Jeff Young.

So the manual grew as the extended community of collaborators grew. Even more, the socialization process that Beck employed in its construction – cultivating in young collaborators a strong feeling that they owned a large stake not only in the manual but in the burgeoning CT enterprise more generally – is evident in the fact that each of the people I interviewed considered themselves central figures, indeed pivotal figures, to the manual's history. Rush made a strong case for that claim. But so did Kovacs:

> I was the only person who wrote it. I mean the original working manual that we had – I was the person who wrote it. I was the person who put it together.

And so did Shaw:

> I was, in my view (subject to what other people remember) really the person who both insisted on writing a manual, who wrote the first 35 pages, who then sent it to John (or to Tim and to John), and then was charged with the main job of writing a manual, writing the cognitive therapy of depression technical parts. So that means all the interventions, describing them in as much detail as we could, and writing what I call the session by session outline, what do you do in the first session, what do you do in the second session, what do you do in the third session.[18]

Rush, Kovacs, and Shaw could each lay claim to having written the manual because Beck relied so heavily on each of their talents and skills. He thought of them – and of all his students over the years who supported cognitive therapy – as extended family.[19]

Understanding Beck's strategy for socializing young, relatively inexperienced therapists into his own neophyte school is central to understanding the power that lay behind CTOD. Beck's entire focus – with the manual just as with everything else – was on socializing his students to join him in thinking differently than psychoanalysts. One of the paradoxes of his manual, then, is that although the explicit purpose was to standardize interventions for a clinical trial, the implicit and far more important agenda was to proselytize and educate in the service of a scientific revolution in psychotherapy.

A particularly salient example of this proselytizing-socializing-revolution-fomenting process appears on the back of a 1975 memorandum to therapists. Most of his therapists in these early years were psychoanalytically oriented. In order for his clinical trial of cognitive therapy to generate viable results, he would need to suspend their psychoanalytic world-view long enough to administer to them a dose of the cognitive one. In other words, he not only had to educate them but also indoctrinate them in the cognitive worldview to ensure that patients would in fact receive cognitive treatments (and not psychoanalytic ones). Hence, the proselytizing and educating:

> In the early interviews, in particular, it is important to construct a 'model' that fits this particular patient. Thus, you ask a question. On the basis of the response, you set up several hypotheses. On the basis of a logical sequence of questions, you verify or modify some hypotheses and discard others. You might, after a series of questions, discard all previous hypotheses and arrive at a new hypothesis. When you feel reasonably confident about your hypothesis, 'try it on' the patient; that is, determine whether *he* thinks it fits and modify it with his help, to get a better fit.[20]

He asked participating therapists to use the manual as a guidebook rather than a cook-book. In this way he was cultivating in them not a blind paint-by-numbers approach but rather a new way of seeing the world, a new set of rules by which to navigate their relationships with their patients and each other. 'In the application of any therapy', he and Rush told therapists in May 1975:

> the therapist operates on the basis of a general outline or theory which he tailors to and utilizes with each specific patient. Thus, the precise specification of therapist behavior or the therapeutic transaction is impossible as patients differ in their presentation, concerns, motivation, etc. On the other hand, therapist behavior is certainly not random. For this reason, this manual moves from the theoretical to the practical, from the general to the specific. It is intended as a guide to the therapist in approaching and interacting therapeutically with the depressed person.[21]

Standardization of treatment was, of course, primary. But Beck assured his therapists that other technologies, like check-lists and ratings of audio- and video-taped sessions, would buttress the manual:

> (w)e are trying to standardize our therapy procedures as much as possible. For research purposes, it is essential that the therapeutic modality be as uniform as possible. This means that the general outline of the treatment manual should be followed but applied in a reasonable, flexible and adaptive way to the specific patient. In order to check on the uniformity of the therapeutic sessions, it is essential that each therapist fill out the 'therapist's check list' at the end of each session. This helps the therapist to stay within the general framework of the cognitive/behavioral therapy and also allows our research analysts an opportunity to check on the 'homogeneity' of the therapy.[22]

With the publication of CTOD in 1979, Beck and his co-authors brought this same proselytizing-socializing-revolution-fomenting process to the general public. Again, the explicit agenda was to lay out the steps of his therapy in a jargon-free, easy-to-follow style. But the implicit agenda was to seduce people away from psychoanalysis (and from other approaches, too, particularly behavior therapy) with the promise that democracy, experimentalism, openness and accountability would prevail, as for example, on page 6: 'In contrast to the more traditional psychotherapies such as psychoanalytic therapy or client-centered therapy, the therapist applying cognitive therapy is continuously active and deliberately interacting with the patient'. And again on p. 7: 'The overall strategy of cognitive therapy may be differentiated from the other schools of therapy by its emphasis on *empirical investigation* of the patient's automatic thoughts, inferences, conclusions, and assumptions. We formulate the patient's dysfunctional idea and beliefs about himself, his experiences, and his future into hypotheses and then attempt to test the validity of these hypotheses in a systematic way. Almost every experience, thus, may provide the opportunity for an experiment relevant to the patient's negative views or beliefs'. The fact that Beck's aim was to cultivate expertise in navigating the world with a new democratic worldview, and not engage solely in paint-by-numbers, is evident again in chapter 11, a verbatim transcript of an interview with a suicidal depressed patient showing how a cognitive therapist 'often has to shift gears and assume a very active role …' and 'draw on his ingenuity'. (p. 225). The fact that the manual outlined in a step-by-step fashion how to do therapy proved enormously exciting to many therapists. But for Beck, outlining those steps was part of a bigger push to teach people how to think like cognitive therapists (and not like psychoanalysts or anyone else).

In sum, CTOD was a manifesto, a public assertion by a new community in a time of new scientific pressures of a new therapeutic order. Beck and his co-authors tethered their revolution to the cognitive revolution in psychology and to Thomas Kuhn's history of science *magnum opus, The Structure of Scientific Revolutions* (Kuhn, 1962). The theme of revolution permeates the book. Some observers of American psychiatry view Beck's CTOD as 'a moment akin to Martin Luther nailing his 95 theses to the Wittenberg church door' (Lieberman, 2015). Beck considers CTOD his 'bible'.

The dissemination of Beck's manual: Gerald Klerman and NIMH

To understand the role of the federal government in furthering Beck's revolution with CTOD we must return to that moment in 1973 when John Rush suggested to Beck that they undertake a clinical trial. In the early 1970s the state of research on the psychotherapy of depression was embryonic. The only psychiatrist doing clinical trials in the psychotherapy of depression was Gerald Klerman, formerly of Yale now of Harvard.

The central narrative here is the relationship Beck built with Klerman. Klerman and Beck together were responsible for ushering in the era of federally funded manualized treatments. Beck had known Klerman through their participation in national conferences on drug research for depression. Klerman's expertise was in the psychopharmacology of depression, but since 1966 he had been using psychotherapy for maintenance treatment once drugs had controlled depressive symptoms. Klerman had hired a social worker at Yale named Myrna Weissman to oversee the psychotherapy component. Their psychotherapy was loosely conceived: derived from Freud but bearing little resemblance to psychoanalysis (Klerman was a lapsed psychoanalytic candidate). They drew inspiration from Harry Stack Sullivan's interpersonal relations theory and from Jerome Frank at Johns Hopkins. They looked at conscious material and solved problems in the here-and-now – in that respect they had much in common with Beck.

On 4 June 1974 Beck asked Klerman about the state of psychotherapy research on depression. Klerman confirmed that most studies were coming out of drug studies:

> Interestingly enough, all these studies were initiated as drug studies, and the psychotherapy was added on. It appears that the psychotherapists in depression have been scandalously reluctant to do outcome studies and that what data we have is only from those studies initiated by persons, like myself, whose initial commitment to therapeutic research began with studies of the efficacy of drugs ...'[23]

Beck and Klerman decided to coordinate their research and began meeting in anticipation of applying for a grant from NIMH for a cooperative study. Klerman made his first visit to Beck's clinic in early 1975. 'I was particularly impressed', he thanked Beck afterward, 'by the high quality of your associates and, also, by the thought and care that has gone into the treatment manual … I think it would be very useful if we could find a way to get together to share techniques and ideas about the treatment of depression'.[24]

Klerman was particularly impressed that Beck included in his manual transcripts (scripts) of patient/therapist interactions. Klerman decided that he should have a similar manual, and asked Weissman to oversee it. '(Gerry) … mentioned that you had a very detailed psychotherapy process manual', she wrote Beck a few weeks later, 'which was used in training therapists for your psychotherapy studies. I'd be interested in seeing a copy as we need to develop a similar procedure[25]'. Beck assured her

> We are in the process of getting the latest edition of our Psychotherapy Treatment Manual typed and I will send a copy on to you as soon as it is ready. I do hope that we can get some kind of a cooperative study going. Since we are working in the same area, it would be a shame not to exchange ideas and also compare or pool data. As we are in the process of gearing up for our major study, it would be good if we could use a research design that is comparable to yours and also use some of the same instruments. If you could send me a copy of your design and instruments, then we will attempt to make our study as synchronous or compatible with yours as possible. I am sure that the National Institute of Mental Health would look favorably upon such a cooperative venture.[26]

Weissman later reflected back on the day Klerman asked her to start writing a manual:

> Gerry gave me Beck's hand-typed manual and he says … 'This manual is terrific and he's written out all these things, he's made scripts …' And I read the manual, and it was, you know, terrific. It was type-written pages and white-outs because they didn't have computers. And (Gerry) said, 'Do this. Good.' So I proceeded to start making a manual.[27]

In the course of writing their manual, Klerman and Weissman decided to call their new approach 'Interpersonal Therapy' (IPT). Beck and Rush paid a visit to the IPT group in Boston in June 1975[28]. Kovacs later made her own trip there to help with their manual[29].

Two more characters enter the story here. Since the late 1960s, NIMH administrators had been trying to convince psychotherapy researchers to undertake clinical trials. But the response had been lukewarm. By the mid-1970s a seasoned NIMH administrator named Morris Parloff and his younger colleague Irene Waskow were intensifying those efforts. In 1976 Beck proposed to Parloff that NIMH fund a one-day conference to coordinate research in the psychotherapy of depression: 'I am afraid that unless there is some coordination', he warned Parloff, 'we will not be able to compare our results or even satisfactorily answer the major questions in this area … I think that the best way to achieve some coordination would be to have a representative group of investigators meet at a convenient place and time to discuss ways of coordinating our work'.[30]

Parloff agreed. [31]Klerman met with Parloff and Waskow at NIMH in July 1976 to discuss the details of the meeting and reported back to Beck that 'the time is propitious for us to discuss the use of common rating scales, criteria for selection of patients, pooling of data, and other matters of common methodology. You are to be congratulated for taking the initiative on bringing us together'.[32] The meeting took place the day before the annual convention of the American Psychological Association on 2 September 1976 in Washington, D.C. The topic was 'An Exploration of the Feasibility of Coordinating Multi-Center Research on the Treatment of Depression'.[33] The group held another meeting in advance of the 1977 SPR meeting in Madison, Wisconsin.[34]

We don't know why exactly Klerman was visiting NIMH in July 1976 but we do know that in October 1977 President Carter nominated him as Administrator of the Alcohol, Drug Abuse and Mental Health Administration (ADAMHA), the parent body of NIMH at the time. [35]As Administrator of ADAMHA, Klerman became the highest ranking psychiatrist making federal mental health policy decisions. Carter tasked Klerman and Congress with evaluating the efficacy and cost-effectiveness of mental health treatments in anticipation of a new national health insurance.

Klerman's priority was to complete the roll-out of an initiative called Treatment Assessment Research (TAR).[36] TAR studied 'the efficacy, safety, and efficiency (cost-effectiveness) of individual techniques or combinations of techniques drawn from within or across treatment modalities'.[37] Klerman's stamp on TAR was unifying psychopharmacology research and psychotherapy research under one institutional umbrella and under one methodology, the RCT: One NIMH branch, one research design, two treatment approaches. In effect, Klerman operationalized psychotherapy as a drug. In so doing, he could now direct federal funds to RCTs comparing drugs with psychotherapy to determine which was most effective with which disorder (Rosner, 2005).

Morris Parloff was responsible for implementing TAR. He jumped on the idea of a multi-center RCT for the treatment of depression. He convinced Klerman to provide $1.3 million out of his Administrator's budget for an NIMH-sponsored multi-site RCT of depression. Parloff appointed Waskow coordinator. The project became known as the Treatment of Depression Collaborative Research Program (TDCRP). TDCRP would compare CT, IPT, a standard drug condition (imipramine plus clinical management) and a control condition. The two therapy manuals would give participating therapists 'the theoretical underpinnings of the approach, the general strategies involved, the major techniques that could be used, and suggestions for dealing with specific problems' (Elkin et al., 1989, p. 972).[38] The manuals would also be the baseline for standardizing treatment 'so that conclusions could be drawn regarding their specific effects' (Elkin et al., 1989, p. 972; Rosner, 2005). Planning began in 1977 and trials were underway by the early 1980s.

Word had already been circulating among NIMH staff about Beck's CT, even before Klerman's arrival in the fall of 1977. One of Beck's former residents was on staff at NIMH. He dispatched a letter to Beck on 28 July 1977 reporting that administrators were excited about CT and the manual:

> I thought you would enjoy the following excerpt from the minutes of a recent Office of the Director meeting discussing treatment assessment research: 'It does seem that really good work will be picked up eventually, when it's well documented. Cognitive therapy with depressed persons being carried about by Aaron Beck and his colleagues at Pennsylvania seems impressive, and seems to be catching on. The work has a very common sense, logical ring to it, and is demonstrable, communicable. They have developed a manual on how to do this kind of therapy. This is being picked up across the country not so much because people are being urged to do this, but because Beck can show the specifics of what is to be done and how they are going about it …'[39]

When the Call For Proposals went out for sites to host TDCRP trials, Beck's and Klerman's manuals became instant national standards for research. The publication of the DSM-III (to which Klerman and Beck were both consultants) in 1980 solidified further the manualized treatment design. NIMH review committees no longer would consider grant proposals unless the research used both a manualized RCT design and DSM-III diagnostic categories.[40]

The rise of manualized psychotherapy protocols was clearly a political process as much as a clinical or scientific one. Beck and Klerman had successfully read the winds of political change at the agency and shifted the courses of their science and practice accordingly. Surely Beck knew that with Klerman now in place at ADAMHA, he was well positioned to reap both economic and political benefits. He and Klerman also were aware that their leadership had succeeded at preserving federal funding for psychotherapy research at a time when the rush of enthusiasm for drugs would have otherwise pushed it out of the market entirely.

Beck also displayed a relentlessness that likely contributed to CTOD reaching a wide readership. Throughout the five years of its construction, Beck insisted on revision after revision after revision from his students. He also was hard-nosed in negotiating a good publishing deal for CTOD with Guilford Press – a new press for whom CTOD would be the first offering. In all these ways Beck's business acumen resulted in CTOD going to press in 1979 – before clinical trials of TDCRP had even begun. By contrast, Klerman and Weissman's manual came out in 1984, a year before Beck's *second* manual – on anxiety (Beck & Emery, 1985) – appeared. And here too, Beck's business sense is in evidence. Klerman and Weissman had gone with Basic Books for their manual. Two other psychotherapy manuals, from Hans Strupp and Lester Luborsky, were also coming out with Basic in 1984 (Klerman, Weissman, Rounsaville, & Chevron, 1984; Luborsky, 1984; Strupp & Binder, 1984). For his anxiety book (1985) Beck left Guilford for Basic.

The sudden appearance of so many manuals in 1984, Parloff later reflected, was one of the 'unintended consequences' of the TDCRP. Very quickly, it seemed, everyone needed manuals: 'The (TDCRP) study set the tone for the review committees because if a new grant came in and it didn't have a manual, the hell with it. If nobody was monitoring whether you really were delivering the therapy you said you were delivering – it became impossible'.[41] In 1982 Waskow (now Elkin) and a colleague convened a two-day workshop at NIMH on 'The Feasibility of Clinical Trials Research on Psychoanalytically Oriented Psychotherapy' to help their psychoanalytic colleagues adapt to this new reality. Strupp's and Luborsky's manuals were products of this very workshop. Such was what Luborsky and DeRubeis called a 'small revolution in psychotherapy research' (Luborsky & DeRubeis, 1984).

The dialectic between clinician and experiment

Despite the rush of enthusiasm for manuals, Parloff remained skeptical about the generalizability of manualized protocols to real-world practice (Rosner, 2005). Parloff, in that sense, was prescient. Ongoing debates over manualized treatments have borne out Parloff's concerns (e.g. Addis et al., 1999; Kazdin, 2008; Parloff, 1998; Silverman,1996; Strupp & Anderson, 1997; Westen & Bradley, 2005; Wilson, 1998).

The question lurking behind these debates is where the locus of clinical authority lies. If the locus lies in quantitative data generated by careful experimentation, and the data show that your treatment works, then you might be confident that your manualized treatment will produce measurable effects in the real world too. If, in contrast, your locus lies in the subjective experience of therapists, then manualized research and practice become problematic. You cannot trust that numbers generated from RCTs will jibe with what you see in the office. You place more trust in a worldview that privileges subjective sensitivity in the moment than objective protocols.

But what if the locus of clinical authority lies somewhere in between? I believe this is the hidden tension in Beck's CTOD revolution. Beck himself has been of two minds about manuals. According to Beck's own recollection of the moment John Rush invited him to undertake a clinical trial in 1973, Rush pitched the argument that no-one would believe that CT worked otherwise:

> There's the famous story that I was teaching cognitive therapy and John (Rush) said, 'You know, this is really great.' And I said, 'Thank you. I agree.' And he said, 'But no one's going to believe you unless you do a clinical trial.' 'Clinical trial? I'll never do a clinical trial. That's back-breaking.' So John said, 'Well, I'll tell you what. I'll do all the framework. I'll do all of this gut work and so on. All you have to do is train the residents in cognitive therapy.' And I said, 'Well, I'm doing that anyhow. Sure.' And so John put it all together and ran the study.[42]

Given Beck's ambition for CT, such a pitch would have been spot-on. And even if Rush hadn't made the pitch just the way Beck remembers it, it is telling that Beck would remember it so. Beck is a savvy businessman, and a successful clinical trial would be the sales-job he needed to convince policy-makers that CT worked. In other words, it would have been completely in keeping with Beck's way of doing business to recognize that CT would have no power in the new RCT marketplace if he couldn't generate positive results with a clinical trial.

At the same time, Beck does not consider CTOD to be a manual. I asked him in 2012 about the history of CTOD as a manual. He answered:

ATB: Basically it isn't a manual. They say it's a manual, but it's got different chapters about different things … It kind of educates the therapist on what to look for and what to do, but it's more educational than descriptive.

RR: You never published the actual manual?

ATB: Well, there wasn't really – we had something way back. John Rush and I put something together and it was sort of manualized, but it was like a three or four page thing.

RR: Oh.

ATB: And then we decided that wasn't the way to go. Although we believed in manualized treatment, I really don't believe in it.

RR: You don't believe in it?

ATB: I believe in it and I don't believe in it [laughing]. I say, you have to have some statement of what people are supposed to do and some way of evaluating what they do. On the other hand, you don't want to restrict the therapist … I rely much more on the education of the therapist to be able to apply the two. So we have something called the Cognitive Therapy Checklist by which we evaluate how well people are doing on various things. So that kind of takes the place of the manual …

RR: So do you think there's a difference between the manual you created and what manualized treatment became?

ATB: Yeah. So for example, if somebody has a phobia and the manual's first session is you talk about what the phobia is, and the second is – say it's a phobia of animals, or cats – you show the person pictures of cats. And then the third is you bring a cat into the room. And then the fourth – that's kind of manualized. It's okay for phobias but for more complex behaviors you can't do that. Because no two people are the same. And even though they have a diagnosis of depression, one person may be so retarded that the best you can do is go out on a walk with him and get him active. And then somebody else is just filled with obsessive thoughts and what we deal with is a kind of a problem-oriented structured approach. And we deal with: What is the problem and how would you tackle that particular problem?

RR: That's very interesting, because you leave a lot of wiggle room for the subjective experience of the therapist.

ATB: You have to. Yeah

So Beck is an experimentalist, but he is also a subjectivist. He seems to be engaged in a complex dance of two world-views which, by the standards of his community, are incommensurate. In focusing on the dialectic between clinician and experiment he is standing squarely in the middle, taking fully neither one side nor the other. The reality of Beck's complicated dance of objectivity and subjectivity, then, displays an epistemological position different from the one for which he is celebrated publicly – raising interesting questions about what Beck actually believes, whether or not (and if not, why not) his publications fully reflect those beliefs, the role that his followers have played in generating and perpetuating positions for which Beck is credited, and Beck's complicity in the perpetuation of those positions.

In 1954 a psychologist at the University of Minnesota named Paul Meehl published a seminal book called *Clinical* vs. *Statistical Prediction* (Meehl, 1954). Meehl argued that statistical prediction would always be more accurate than clinical (subjective) prediction. And yet Meehl frequently and deliberately engaged, in private, in generous unanchored speculations, often of a psychoanalytic nature. His attraction to psychoanalysis was strong and he kept a picture of Freud on his office wall. Meehl and Beck enjoyed a correspondence in the late 1960s. Meehl explained to Beck that:

> I favor cultivating maximum freedom in theoretical speculation, and I feel no particular obligation to present positive confirming evidence when I propound my theoretical concept. What preserves this attitude from resulting in Freudian metaphysics is the Popperian insistence upon tightening up the theoretical network sufficiently to permit strong discorroboration by negative findings … It is important that you understand this methodological frame of reference, which permits a 'Minnesota dustbowl empiricist' (on <u>certain</u> issues) to cerebrate so free-wheelingly on others.[43]

To which Beck replied,

> After reading [Meehl's article with Cronbach on Construct Validity, 1957], I experienced a sudden enlightenment and started on the road of searching for more empirical data to support psychoanalytic constructs. As time went on, I realized that support for these postulates was ultimately derived from the declarative statements of the psychoanalytic authorities rather than from evidence; I began to quaver in my belief that '20,000 analysts can't be wrong.' Ever since that time, primarily as a result of reading the research literature and doing some research myself, I have moved much closer to the position of 'the dustbowl empiricist'.[44]

Meehl reconciled these oppositions by trying to tame his subjectivity (grounded in his psychoanalytic training) through the Popperian discipline of disconfirmation. Beck made a similar bargain: he tried to bracket his subjectivity (grounded in his psychoanalytic training) into an empirical frame of reference. Beck and Meehl were grappling with the same challenge of bridging experimentalism and subjectivism that the therapists in the three NIMH-sponsored psychotherapy conferences in the 1960s faced – which suggests that the CTOD revolution may not have been as decisive a victory for experimentalists as generally understood, even for the man whose own work sparked that revolution.

Conclusion

Beck's manualized-protocol revolution was over two decades in the making. Even then, Beck's own personal star didn't really reach its zenith until the late 1990s, with the rise of Evidence-Based Medicine (EBM). The full history of EBM has yet to be written, but recent versions of its origin story (see Smith & Rennie, 2014) tell us that EBM, just like the DSM-III and Beck's CTOD, was a response to the same challenge physicians faced following the Kefauver-Harris amendment of 1962 and Carter's push for national health insurance in the late 1970s. For 30 years, physicians grappled with shifting their locus of clinical judgment from the subjective wisdom of the individual doctor to the promise of the statistical aggregate from clinical trials. Born out of the same moment, and championing the same basic principles, Beck and Klerman's manualized-protocol revolution and EBM were destined to dovetail.

What is sometimes lost in this era of EBM, however, is that CTOD was, at its center, a very personal response to a crisis in Beck's psychoanalytic community that nearly did him in professionally. So, certainly the manualized therapy revolution did solve the problem of getting psychotherapy into the RCT game and providing congress and insurance companies quantitative proof of therapy's efficacy and cost-effectiveness. But for Beck personally, CTOD was really a totem – a bible, as he calls it – of everything that had gone wrong with psychoanalysis politically and everything he was promising himself (and his community) would now go right. Far from employing it solely as a mechanical instrument, Beck played CTOD as a trumpet of democracy, openness, accountability, skeptical inquiry, and self-determination. And embedded deeply within it remains the kernel of subjectivity. These are not objective phenomena. They are values, virtues. They are beliefs – which are about as subjective as one can be. And so even in the era of objectivity in psychotherapy research, the press of the subjective within it remains strong.[45] The problem at the heart of those three NIMH-sponsored psychotherapy research conferences in the 1960s, it seems, remains to be solved.

Notes

1. To achieve scientific 'legitimacy' had in fact been the aim since the late 1960s of some North American psychotherapy researchers, many affiliated with the Society for Psychotherapy Research (SPR).
2. Paul's *Insight vs. Desensitization* was the first published manual. Most behavior therapy manuals, however, remained unpublished. See also author's telephone interview with Marvin Goldfried, 24 November 2015.
3. See Andrew Gerber, conversation with the author, October 2015.
4. Transcript of an interview with Aaron T. Beck/Interviewer Marjorie Weishaar, 4 August 1991.
5. Author's interview with John Rush, 16 October 2013, Philadelphia, PA; Author's interview with Jim Stinnette, 17 October 2013, Philadelphia, PA.

6. Anonymous, undated 'Cognitive-Behavioral Treatment Program for Depression', Mood Clinic, 9 Gates, HUP. Personal Collection, Aaron T. Beck.
7. Author's interview with John Rush, October 16, 2013. Beck's colleagues, students and friends call him 'Tim.' See also Rush, Khatami, & Beck, 1975.
8. 'Protocol for Cognitive Behavioral Therapy of Depression', 12 October 1973, rough draft. Personal Collection, ATB. The author thanks Dr. Aaron T. Beck for granting access to, and permission to quote from, his personal collection.
9. Personal Collection, Aaron T. Beck.
10. See within this article the reference to 'A. T. Beck, A. J. Rush and M. Kovacs, *Individual treatment manual for cognitive/behavioral psychotherapy of depression*. Unpublished manuscript, 1975. Available from Dr. Aaron T. Beck, 429 Stouffer Building, Philadelphia General Hospital, Philadelphia, Pennsylvania 19104'.
11. Author's interview with David M. Clark, November 20, 2014, Philadelphia, PA.
12. Beck and Rush wrote in a June 1974 draft, for instance, that '(the therapist) needs to sound out the patient and reach a consensus on which problem(s) to tackle first and what methods to use'. Aaron T. Beck and John Rush, 1974, 'The treatment manual for cognitive-behavioral therapy of depression', p. 7, Personal Collection, Aaron T. Beck.
13. ATB to John Paul Brady, 23 October 1974, Personal Collection, Aaron T. Beck.
14. 'Protocol for the development of a cognitive-behavioral (C/B) therapy study for treating depression and anxiety, August 1974,' p. 3 Personal Collection, Aaron T. Beck.
15. Author's telephone interview with Maria Kovacs, July 18, 2013.
16. AT Beck and AJ Rush, 'The treatment manual for cognitive-behavioral therapy of depression', June, 1974; AT Beck and AJ Rush, 'Cognitive Behavioral Therapy of Depression: Treatment Manual', 14 May 1975; AJ Rush, AT Beck, M Kovacs, M Khatami, R Fitzgibbons, and T Wolman, 'Comparison of cognitive and pharmacotherapy in depressed outpatients: A preliminary report'. Personal Collection, Aaron T. Beck.
17. Author's interview with Brian Shaw, June 12, 2013, Toronto, Ontario, Canada.
18. Author's interview with John Rush, October 16, 2013, Philadelphia, PA; Author's telephone interview with Marika Kovacs, July 18, 2013; Author's interview with Brian Shaw, June 12, 2013 Toronto, Ontario, Canada.
19. He kept a file in his personal papers labeled 'Extended Family' containing lists of the many students he had trained and of researchers with whom he shared common purpose.
20. AT Beck, Memorandum to the psychotherapists participating in the depression therapy project (rough draft 2/24/75). Personal Collection, Aaron T. Beck.
21. AT Beck and AJ Rush 'Treatment Manual for Cognitive-Behavioral Therapy of Depression, Revision 5/14/75', p. 1. Personal Collection, Aaron T. Beck.
22. ATB, 'Memorandum to psychotherapists in depression therapy project,' rough draft 2/24/75. Personal Collection, Aaron T. Beck.
23. GLK to ATB, 18 June 1974, Personal Collection, Aaron T. Beck.
24. GLK to ATB, 6 February 1975, Personal Collection, Aaron T. Beck.
25. MMW to ATB, 20 February 1975, Personal Collection, Aaron T. Beck.
26. ATB to MMW, March 5, 1975, Personal Collection Aaron T. Beck; ATB to GK, March 5, 1975, Personal Collection Aaron T. Beck.
27. Author's interview with Myrna M. Weissman, December 23, 2014, New York, New York.
28. GLK to ATB, 23 June 1975, Personal Collection Aaron T. Beck.

29. Author's telephone interview with Marika Kovacs, 18 July 2013; Author's interview with A. John Rush, 16 October 2013, Philadelphia, PA.
30. ATB to MBP, 29 June 1976. Personal Collection, Aaron T. Beck.
31. IEW to ATB, 16 August 1976. Personal Collection, Aaron T. Beck.
32. GK to ATB, 22 July 1976. Personal Collection, Aaron T. Beck.
33. Agenda, 2 September 1976. Personal Collection, Aaron T. Beck.
34. ATB to Steve Hollon, 18 March 1977. Personal Collection, Aaron T. Beck.
35. Jimmy Carter: 'Alcohol, Drug Abuse, and Mental Health Administration Nomination of Gerald L. Klerman To Be Administrator'. 12 October 1977. Online by Gerhard Peters and John T. Woolley, *The American Presidency Project*. http://www.presidency.ucsb.edu/ws/?pid=6784
36. James Isbister, the Administrator of ADAMHA in 1975, initiated TAR as a working group across the three institutes of the National Institutes of Health. Klerman expanded its scope.
37. Minutes, 119th meeting of the National Advisory Mental Health Council (p. 13) (6–7 December 1979). Department of Health, Education and Welfare, Public Health Service, ADAMHA, NIMH.
38. Memorandum from Chief, Psychotherapy and Behavioral Interventions Section of the Clinical Research Branch, to Director, National Institute of Mental Health (15 July 1980). Personal collection of Barry E. Wolfe.
39. Stephen P. Hersh to ATB, July 28, 1977. Personal Collection, Aaron T. Beck.
40. Author's interview with Barry Wolf, Baltimore, MD, 24 March 2001.
41. Author's interview with Morris Parloff, 21 March 2001.
42. Author's interview with Aaron T. Beck, spring 2012.
43. PEM to ATB, February 26, 1968, Personal Collection, Aaron T. Beck. See also Meehl's preface to the 1996 edition of *Clinical* versus *Statistical Prediction* (New York: Jason Aronson) in which he admits that the book was an attempt to grapple publicly with his commitment to both worldviews.
44. ATB to PEM, March 13, 1968, Personal Collection, Aaron T. Beck.
45. See, for instance, Gaudiano, 2013

Disclosure statement

No potential conflict of interest was reported by the author.

References

Addis, M. E., Wade, W. A., & Hatgis, C. (1999). Barriers to dissemination of evidence-based practices: Addressing practitioners' concerns about manual-based psychotherapies. *Clinical Psychology: Science and Practice, 6*(4), 430–441.

Barlow, D. H., & Greene, K. A. I. (2001). Clinical psychology: Manual-based treatment. *International Encyclopedia of the Social and Behavioral Sciences, 5*(2), 2036–2040.

Beck, A. T. (1963). Thinking and depression I: Idiosyncratic content and cognitive distortions. *Archives of General Psychiatry, 9,* 324–333.

Beck, A. T. (1964). Thinking and depression II: Theory and therapy. *Archives of General Psychiatry, 10,* 561–571.

Beck, A. T. (1967). *Depression: clinical, experimental and theoretical aspects.* New York, NY: Hoeber Medical Division, Harper & Row.

Beck, A. T., & Emery, G. (1985). *Anxiety disorders and phobias: A cognitive approach.* New York, NY: Basic Books.

Beck, A. T., Rush, A. J., Shaw, B. J., & Emery, G. (1979). *Cognitive therapy of depression.* New York, NY: Guilford Press.

Bergin, A. E., & Strupp, H. H. (1972). *Changing frontiers in the Science of psychotherapy.* Chicago, IL: Aldine Atherton.

Bothwell, L. A., Greene, J. A., Podolsky, S. H., & Jones, S. D. (2016). Assessing the gold standard – Lessons from the history of RCTs. *New England Journal of Medicine, 374,* 2175–2181.

Dobson, K. S., & Shaw, B. F. (1988). The use of treatment manuals in cognitive therapy: Experience and issues. *Journal of Consulting and Clinical Psychology, 56*(5), 673–680 (p. 674).

Elkin, I., Shea, T., Watkins, J. T., Imber, S. D., Sotsky, S. M., Collins, J. F., … Parloff, M. B. (1989). National institute of mental health treatment of depression collaborative research program: General effectiveness of treatments. *Archives of General Psychiatry, 46,* 971–983.

Fiske, D. W., Hunt, H. F., Luborsky, L., Orne, M. T., Parloff, M. B., Reiser, M. F., & Tuma, A. H. (1970). Planning of research on effectiveness in psychotherapy. *American Psychologist, 25,* 727–737. Published simultaneously in *Archives of General Psychiatry*, 22(1), 22–32.

Gaudiano, B. A. (2013, September 30). Psychotherapy's image problem. *New York Times,* A25.

Greene, J. A., & Podolsky, S. H. (2012). Reform, regulation, and pharmaceuticals – The Kefauver–Harris amendments at 50. *New England Journal of Medicine, 367,* 1481–1483.

Hale, N. G. (1995). *The rise and crisis of psychoanalysis in the United States: Freud and the Americans, 1917–1985.* New York, NY: Oxford University Press.

Jones, D. S. (2000). Visions of a cure: Visualization, clinical trials, and controversies in cardiac therapeutics, 1968–1998. *Isis, 91,* 504–541.

Kazdin, A. E. (2008). Evidence-based treatment and practice. *American Psychologist, 63*(6), 146–159.

Klerman, G. K., Weissman, M. M., Rounsaville, B. J., & Chevron, E. S. (1984). *Interpersonal psychotherapy of depression.* New York, NY: Basic Books.

Kuhn, T. (1962). *The structure of scientific revolution.* Chicago, IL: University of Chicago Press.

Latour, B. (1987). *Science in action: How to follow scientists and engineers through society.* Cambridge, MA: Harvard University Press.

Lieberman, J. A. (2015). *Shrinks: The untold story of psychiatry.* New York, NY: Little, Brown & Company.

Luborsky, L. (1984). *Principles of psychoanalytic psychotherapy: A manual for supportive-expressive treatment.* New York, NY: Basic Books.

Luborsky, L., & DeRubeis, R. J. (1984). The use of psychotherapy treatment manuals: A small revolution in psychotherapy research style. *Clinical Psychology Review, 4,* 5–14.

Marks, H. (1997). *The progress of experiment: Science and therapeutic reform in the United States, 1900–1990.* Cambridge: Cambridge University Press.

Meehl, P. (1954). *Clinical versus statistical prediction*. Minneapolis: University of Minnesota Press.

Parloff, M. B. (1979). Can psychotherapy research guide the policymaker? *American Psychologist, 34*, 296–306.

Parloff, M. B. (1998). Is psychotherapy more than manual labor? *Clinical Psychology: Science and Practice, 5*(3), 376–381.

Paul, G. L. (1966). *Insight vs. desensitization in psychotherapy*. Stanford: Stanford University Press.

Rosner, R. I. (2005). Psychotherapy research and the National Institute of Mental Health, 1948–1980. In W. E. Pickren & S. F. Schneider (Eds.), *Psychology and the National Institute of Mental Health* (pp. 113–150). Washington, DC: American Psychological Association.

Rosner, R. I. (2012). Aaron T. Beck's drawings and the psychoanalytic origin story of cognitive therapy. *History of Psychology, 15*(1), 1–18.

Rosner, R. I. (2014). The splendid isolation of Aaron T. Beck. *Isis, 105*(4), 734–758.

Rush, A. J., Beck, A. T., Kovacs, M., & Hollon, S. (1977). Comparative efficacy of cognitive therapy and pharmacotherapy in the treatment of depressed outpatients. *Cognitive Therapy and Research, 1*(1), 17–37.

Rush, A. J., Khatami, M., & Beck, A. T. (1975). Cognitive and behavior therapy in chronic depression. *Behavior Therapy, 6*, 398–404.

Silverman, W. H. (1996). Cookbooks, manuals, and paint-by-numbers: Psychotherapy in the 90's. *Psychotherapy: Theory, Research, Practice Training, 33*(2), 207–215.

Smith, R., & Rennie, D. (2014). Evidence-based medicine – An oral history. *Journal of the American Medical Association, 311*(4), 365–367.

Strupp, H. H., & Anderson, T. (1997). On the limitations of therapy manuals. *Clinical Psychology: Science and Practice, 4*(1), 76–82.

Strupp, H. H., & Binder, J. L. (1984). *Psychotherapy in a new key: A Guide to time-limited dynamic psychotherapy*. New York, NY: Basic Books.

Westen, D., & Bradley, R. (2005). Empirically supported complexity: Rethinking evidence-based practice in psychotherapy. *Current Directions in Psychological Science, 14*(5), 266–271.

Wilson, G. T. (1998). Manual based treatment and clinical practice. *Clinical Psychology: Science and Practice, 5*(3), 363–375.

Modernist Pills against Brazilian Alienism (1920–1945)

Cristiana Facchinetti ⓘ

ABSTRACT

Psychoanalysis arrived in Brazil at the turn of the twentieth century and was frequently used as a new tool in the process of conservative modernization. As such, it was used by psychiatrists, eugenicists and hygienists in their projects. But avant-garde Brazilian writers appropriated it in a different manner. They saw psychoanalysis as a new form of cultural therapy that represented the new Brazilian 'modernity'. The paper deals precisely with this project. With this aim in mind, it analyses several works of the leading authors of the Modernist Movement and their Manifestos, seeking to draw attention to the particular way in which psychoanalysis was appropriated as a psychotherapeutic tool capable of assisting in the creation of an identity for the country. For this analysis, the concept of circulation and of appropriation were chosen as theoretical reference.

PILDORAS MODERNISTAS CONTRA LA ALIENACION

El Psicoanálisis llegó a Brasil a principios del siglo XX y fue utilizado frecuentemente como un nuevo instrumento en el proceso de modernización conservadora. Como tal fue la provincia de psiquiatras, eugenistas e higienistas en sus proyectos. Sin embargo, los escritoires brasileros se apropiaron de él de una manera diferente, viendo el Psicoanálisis como una nueva forma de terapia cultural que representaba la nueva 'modernidad' brasilera. Este artículo trata precisamente de ese proyecto y con esta meta en mente, analiza varios trabajos de destacados autores del movimiento Modernista y sus Manifiestos, buscando llamar la atención hacia la manera particular en la cual el Psicoaálisis fue tomado como un instrument terapéutico capaz de ayudar a la creación de una identidad para el país. Se ha escogido los conceptos de circulación y de apropiación como referencia teórica.

Pillole moderniste contro l'alienismo brasiliano

La psicoanalisi arrivò in Brasile a cavallo del ventesimo secolo e fu spesso utilizzata come nuovo strumento nel processo di una modernizzazione conservatrice. Come tale, è stata usata da psichiatri, eugenisti e igienisti nei loro progetti. Tuttavia gli scrittori brasiliani d'avanguardia se ne sono appropriati in un modo diverso. Videro la psicoanalisi come una nuova forma di terapia culturale che rappresentava la nuova 'modernità' brasiliana. Il presente articolo tratta precisamente di questo progetto. Per perseguire questo obiettivo, analizza diverse opere dei principali autori del Movimento Modernista e dei loro seguaci, cercando di attirare l'attenzione sul modo in cui ci si è appropriati della psicoanalisi quale strumento psicoterapeutico in grado di supportare la creazione di un'identità nazionale. A tal fine, il concetto di circolazione e appropriazione è stato scelto come riferimento teorico.

Des pilules modernistes contre l'aliénisme brésilien

La psychanalyse est arrivée au Brésil au tournant du 20ième siècle et était fréquemment utilisée comme l'outil novateur d'une modernisation conservatrice. À ce titre elle était utilisée dans les projets de psychiatres, d'eugénistes et d'hygiénistes. Cependant les écrivains avant-gardistes se la sont appropriée différemment. Ils ont vu dans la psychanalyse une forme nouvelle de thérapie culturelle représentant la nouvelle « modernité » brésilienne. Cet article explore très précisément ce projet. Avec cet objectif en tête, il analyse plusieurs travaux d'auteurs phares du Mouvement Moderniste ainsi que leurs Manifestes, cherchant à attirer l'attention sur la façon particulière dont la psychanalyse a été transformée en un outil psychothérapeutique capable d'aider à la création de l'identité de la nation. Pour cette analyse le concept de circulation et d'appropriation a été choisi comme référence théorique.

Μοντέρνα Χάπια ενάντια στην Βραζιλιάνικη Ψυχιατρική

Περίληψη: Η ψυχανάλυση έφτασε στη Βραζιλία στις απαρχές του 20ου αιώνα και συχνά χρησιμοποιήθηκε ως ένα νέο εργαλείο στη διαδικασία του συντηρητικού εκσυγχρονισμού. Ως τέτοιο, χρησιμοποιήθηκε από ψυχιάτρους, ευγονικούς και υγιεινολόγους στο έργο τους. Από την άλλη πλευρά, πρωτοποριακοί Βραζιλιάνοι συγγραφείς χρησιμοποίησαν την ψυχανάλυση με έναν διαφορετικό τρόπο. Αντιμετώπισαν την ψυχανάλυση ως μια νέα μορφή πολιτισμικής θεραπείας που αντιπροσώπευε το νέο Βραζιλιάνικο Νεωτερικότητα. Αυτό το άρθρο ασχολείται ακριβώς με αυτό το έργο. Με αυτό τον στόχο, αναλύει διάφορα έργα των κύριων συγγραφέων της Νεωτερικότητας και των διακηρύξεων τους, αποσκοπώντας να αναδείξει τον συγκεκριμένο τρόπο με τον οποίο η ψυχανάλυση χρησιμοποιήθηκε ως ένα ψυχοθεραπευτικό εργαλείο το οποίο μπορούσε να συμβάλει στη δημιουργία ταυτότητας για τη χώρα. Για αυτή την ανάλυση, οι έννοιες της κυκλοφορίας και της σφετερισμού επιλέχθηκαν ως το θεωρητικό πλαίσιο.

Some historians claim that psychoanalysis surfaced in Brazil from the late nineteenth century onwards. According to these sources, Juliano Moreira[1] gave lectures on the subject as professor in Bahia in 1899. Others place the ground zero of its dissemination in the first doctoral thesis on the subject in 1914, at Rio de Janeiro's School of Medicine. These references point to the realization of the use of psychoanalysis as a therapeutic tool in the Chair of Psychiatry at the School of Medicine and in the National Hospice of the Alienated. Other authors draw attention to the dissemination of psychoanalysis in the 1920s, linked to hygienist and eugenicist principles (Facchinetti & Castro, 2015a). These actions contributed to psychoanalysis being interpreted as a correctional tool for individuals and the nation as a whole. Thus, psychoanalysis came to be disseminated in the fields of work, education and re-socialization.

However, psychoanalysis did not only fulfil the objectives of this conservative modernization. Avant-garde writers used experimental aesthetics in addition to psychoanalysis to place their bets on cultural therapy that could offer an iconic image of a brand new modern identity for the country. This is essentially the scope of this article.

1. The others

Although the Americas are at the core of modern ideals, their initial participation in the 'concert of nations' was decidedly gauche. In the words of travellers of the period, such as Cornelius de Pauw, nature took 'everything from one hemisphere of the globe to give it to the other': on the one hand, humanity, and on the other, ' stupidity (…)' (as cited in Laplantine, 2000, p. 44).

Thus, since the beginning of Brazilian colonization, its indigenous people and climate were perceived as being an obstacle to the 'spontaneous and natural' tendencies of the historical development of societies (Sallas, 2010). Based on a Eurocentric standpoint, modern sciences also forged the 'neutral' and 'rational' concept of different evolutionary levels of human societies, distinguishing 'civilized' European societies from others, understood as belonging to the most primitive level of savagery or even barbarism (Lander, 2005, pp. 21–53). As Freud described it, the encounter with the *Other* left deep impressions on Enlightenment thinking:

> When I speak of disillusionment, everyone will know at once what I mean. (…) We were prepared to find that wars between the primitive and the civilized people, between the races who are divided by the colour of their skin (…) would occupy mankind for some time to come. But we permitted ourselves to have other hopes. We had expected the great world-dominating nations of white race upon whom

the leadership of the human species has fallen, who were known to have world-wide interests as their concern, to whose creative powers were due not only our technical advances towards the control of nature but the artistic and scientific standards of civilization - we had expected these people to succeed in discovering another way of settling misunderstandings and conflicts of interest. (…) But the great nations themselves, it might have been supposed, would have acquired so much comprehension of what they had in common, and so much tolerance for their differences, that 'foreigner' and 'enemy' could no longer be merged, as they still were in classical antiquity, into a single concept. (Freud, 1915a/2009, pp. 5, 6)

However, the principles of progress and evolution were not sufficient to ensure dignified social conditions for all human beings. On the contrary, the process of modernization was the stage for growing social malaise and of criticism against the capitalist model of society. Gradually, suspicions about the theses of individual autonomy, sovereignty, evolution and progress were voiced (Ricoeur, 1988).

This 'critical consciousness' was a revolutionary tendency that became known as Modernism (Birman, 2000) and rallied part of the philosophical, political, literary and artistic counter-discourse of European Modernity. Among its 'prophets', Nietzsche, Marx and Freud (Andrade, 1929/1992) emphasized their disquiet and discomfort with modernity. According to this line of thinking, what was then considered the apex of civilization, namely Europe, was in a state of decadence and sundry internal contradictions existed in its very core. There was growing suspicion that Europeans '(…) had never risen as high as we thought' (Freud, 1915b/1986; p. 15). The crisis became even more acute after World War I, when 'the Great Depression confirmed the belief of intellectuals, activists, and ordinary citizens that there was something fundamentally wrong with the world they lived in' (Hobsbawm, 1995, p. 98).

Therefore, the former optimism about progress was the 'victim of the internal contradictions of its advance' (Hobsbawm, 1995, p. 25). The cards were shuffled, and the castle of evolutionary concepts collapsed. It was no longer possible to affirm, at least without blinking, ontological differences between civilization and barbarism (Freud, 1933/1986), as Freud stated:

We cannot but feel that no event has ever destroyed so much that is precious in the common possessions of humanity, confused so many of the clearest intelligences, or so thoroughly debased what is highest. Science herself has lost her passionless impartiality; her deeply embittered servants seek for weapons from her with which to contribute towards the struggle with the enemy. Anthropologists feel driven to declare that enemy inferior and degenerate, psychiatrists issue a diagnosis of his disease of mind or spirit. (Freud, 1915a/2009, p. 4)

The crisis affected many European intellectuals of the period. Among them, the literary avant-garde began calling into question the model of a single civilization as the apex of an evolutionary linearity. In this process, literature was used as a source for the expression of new sensitivities. This was also the case with psychoanalysis, which served as an instrument to turn the civilizing model onto its head:

> Psycho-analysis has inferred (…) that the primitive, savage and evil impulses of mankind have not vanished in any of its individual members, but persist, although in a repressed state, in the unconscious (…) and lie in wait for opportunities of becoming active once more. It has further taught us that our intellect is a (…) plaything and tool of our instincts and affects (…). (Freud, 1915b/1986, p. 340)

If barbarism and primitivism were present in all mankind, and if the European civilizing model had demanded more than it was possible for men to endure, provoking the eruption of destructive forces of such magnitude, it was necessary to return to the starting point, namely to the primitive, then 'hidden in the interior of the individual' (Russo, 2002). This was what Dadaism, Surrealism and Expressionism did (Bradbury & McFarlane, 1989, p. 31), for example.

2. Modernist therapy

Since the nineteenth century, impacted by what was then considered the decadence of European civilization, primitivist artists such as Paul Gauguin (1848–1903) came to value the simplicity of *naif* art of non-Western peoples (Rhodes, 1994).

After World War I, primitivism gained a new impetus, defining itself in contrast to the decadence of Europe. But instead of just revisiting *barbaric* art, the solution of a different model of culture also emerged as valid at an aesthetic level, as can be seen in the Portuguese poetry of Fernando Pessoa,[2] who affirmed:

> True modern art has to be totally denationalized – to accumulate within itself all parts of the world (…). And, once this fusion is spontaneously completed, it will result in art-of-all-arts, a spontaneously complex inspiration. (Pessoa, 1998, p. 408)

But, whilst in the European context modernity was located between the European and the 'primitive', on the other side of the globe, in Latin America, the 'primitive' came to be understood as the pre-colonial past. The avant-garde used it both to propose aesthetic reformulations and to place it in a 'prehistory' pushed into the background by European civilization. In this sense, primitivism was linked to the very concept of modernity, with a certain equivalence between modernism and primitivism (Mata, 2013; p. 20). It was from this new perspective that Brazil emerged as a type of cultural experiment that could contribute to the 'concert of the nations'. Thus, while the European avant-garde sought to denationalize itself to break with its artificial model of civilization in order to accumulate in itself 'all parts of the world' (Pessoa, 1998, p. 114), Brazilian modernists came to assert that the fusion of differences had already occurred in Brazil and was waiting to be recognized and valued as such. The concept of miscegenation ceased to represent degeneracy and came to indicate a unique ability to produce a cultural synthesis of differences.

Thus, the psycho-diagnosis established by the avant-garde was that our alienation had been produced by our persistent desire to catch up with the others. To recover, it was necessary to free 'Homo Brasiliensis' from the chains imposed by

'European culture that was rotten to the core' (*Revista de Antropofagia* – second edition, 1975).

When the *Group of Five*[3] got together to organize Brazil's Modern Art Week (São Paulo, 1922), the members converged on a variant influenced by futurism, which favoured the modern reality over the imperial and colonized past, in the aesthetic quest for a new language to transcend what 'had gone before' (Santiago, 2000, p. 15). But as shown in the *Pau-Brasil* Manifesto (1924), this issue was swiftly abandoned:

> The work of the futurist generation was cyclopic.
>
> To adjust the empire clock of national literature.
>
> Once this step is completed, the problem is different.
>
> To be regional and pure in our era.
>
> (Andrade, O., 2001, p.65)

Thus, the 'Brazilian way of being' became a central issue in the therapeutic-aesthetic program, as did the notion of primitivism, both thought to help in the formulation of a new model to re-launch its subjectivity different from the Western model.

In assuming the primitive as Brazil's unconscious, modernist therapy began to seek the cure for local alienation through the acknowledgement of the previously repressed components of identity, with a view to producing a narrative capable of altering local and regional consciousness and redeeming the latent contents considered to be the popular and characteristic mnemonic traits of the country.

In this process, concepts derived from psychoanalytic theory began to circulate among these authors in the redemption of historical legacies, with the objective of 'liberating the most diverse historical, social, aesthetic and ethnic repressed aspects of the country' (Facchinetti, 2003).

The 'redemption of repressed aspects' or 'the reaction against all the negative aspects of tradition' was initially instituted to make it possible to recover the 'parameters' of popular tradition 'forgotten in the present' as a way to (re) discover Brazil through symbolic appropriation and invention (Birman, 2009).

The amnesia, considered as a negative aspect of European colonialism, and intrinsically linked to it as a commitment to the symptoms of classical literature, could be overcome by the recovery of the mnemonic traits of local culture (Facchinetti, 2012, p. 53). This was the way modernists sought to (re) create Brazilian identity: the healing of its alienation could come from keeping alive the tension between self-recognition with its 'improvised solutions' (Andrade, 1992, p. 15), absorbing the cultural divisions, partialities and multiplicities in a heterogeneous composition that prevented the realization of their essence.

3. A case study

In one of the famous assessments of Modernism made in the 1940s, Oswald de Andrade[4] established a parallel between the movement of the Minas Gerais separatist conspiracy (1789)[5] and the Modern Art Week of 1922, considering both movements as attempts to put Brazil in line with other civilized nations (Andrade, 1991). According to him, it began with Mário de Andrade's *'Prefácio Interessantíssimo'* (Andrade, 1922/1987) and was then encapsulated in the 'Pau-Brasil' Manifesto (Andrade, 2001). Both pieces together composed this national model that brought together the 'general tendencies' that Mário de Andrade[6] had talked about (Andrade, 1992, p. 15).

The collection of verses, also called *Pau-Brasil* (Andrade, O., 2001), reaffirmed native primitivism as being central to the movement. In fact, Oswald later considered it to be the 'only finding of 1922' (Andrade, 1991; p. 111). Thus, primitivism was considered a Brazilian 'theory of culture' and, at the same time, as a treatment for the re-education of local sensitivities (Nunes, 1978). The idea was to purge the European 'literacy plague' (Prado, 1924/1990; pp. 289, 290). The cure was to be the Brazilian language, 'The way we speak is the way we are' (Andrade, 2001).

Mario de Andrade enthusiastically adhered to the 'Pau-Brasil' program (Andrade, M., 1924/1975, p. 369). Therefore, he proposed to write 'foolish language, naive thought, only to call the attention of the strongest (…) to this weak and indecisive monster that is Brazil' (Andrade, M., 1924/1975, p. 370). His primitivism was at its peak in *Macunaíma* (Andrade, 1928/1993), marked by an experimental and popular, but complex and synthesizing *Brazilianness*, in which the jungle and industry, the indigenous and the Portuguese, as well as the highest technologies would meet, forming the 'Tupi' composite of the 1920s.

> In the depths of the virgin bush Macunaíma, the hero of our people, was born. He was black as pitch, the son of the dead of night. There was a moment when the silence was so great, listening to the burbling of the Uraricoera river that Tapanhumas [a tribal Indian] gave birth to an ugly child. This is the child that they called Macunaíma. (Andrade, 1928/1993, p. 9)

The story begins in the wilderness, passes through different regions of Brazil and ends with the return of Macunaíma to the hinterlands. During his travels, the hero changes continuously due to his contact with civilization, while also modifying it, in a world in which the *self* and the *Other* interact, merge and transform each other by assimilation. It is in this way that his return to the backlands, at the end of the novel, is the moment of this incorporation. The character transcends frontiers and territories, mixes races and customs and gives new meanings to history, 'deconstructing the stereotypes based on the existence of a Brazilian essence' (Bernd, 1992, pp. 47–50). Being the synthesis of incessant metamorphoses, virtues, defects, different ethnicities and different cultures, Macunaíma unites the primitive and the civilized, 'the hinterlands and the school' (Andrade, 2001), by means of an identity in the process of formation (Martins, 2006; pp. 12, 13). In the end, we are left with the tragic portrait of a man 'without qualities' (Facchinetti, 2003; p. 137) as the 'national icon' (Moraes, 2004, p. 4), strongly praised by Oswald. After all, from his point of view, this was the direction the modernist movement had to follow from then on:

> The rehabilitation of the primitive is a task for the Americans. Everyone knows the depressing concept that the Europeans used for colonizing purposes. [...] I consider it essential to rethink concepts regarding Homo Americanus. I appeal to all scholars of this great subject to take into consideration the greatness of the primitive, its solid concept of life as "devouring", and project an entire philosophy in the making. (Andrade, 1929/1992, pp. 231, 232)

But Macunaíma was the last major work in which the literary and mainly political ambitions of Mario and Oswald de Andrade coincided: the criticisms against the Pau-Brasil Movement and its primitivism grew along with the conservative trends of the late 1920s (Boaventura, 1995), dividing the modernists. Mário and Oswald finally parted company in 1929:

> (...) if [Macunaíma] was written in fun, the rereading of the book began to distress me profoundly. Today it seems to me to be a perverse satire. Indeed, it is so perverse that I no longer believe that habits and customs can be corrected through satire. (Andrade, 1929/1968, p. 58)

From then onwards, Mário de Andrade distanced himself from deconstructivism. This was undoubtedly due to his political militancy and his intention to participate in the formulation of proposals for a 'critical construction of the Brazil file' opting for the 'death of the poet' in the name of the foundation of 'Brazilianness as a tradition' (Birman, 2009, p. 197).

As was the case with the entire Latin American avant-garde generation, Mário de Andrade was also divided between the possibility of expanding a poetic practice that was creative and respectful of his own individuality and the need to articulate this poetic practice to a stratified and dependent society in order to champion the process of social transformation. 'This situation fuelled the terrible contradictions between the artistic demand for freedom and the political responsibility of an art of circumstance' (Antelo, 1986, p. 33).

A year after the Andrades parted company, Brazil suffered a coup. When Getulio Vargas came to lead the provisional government in 1930, he co-opted intellectuals to conceive a model of modernization for the country and to participate in actions under his leadership. Although Mário de Andrade was initially left wing, he later collaborated with the government for the implementation of new models of culture and education.

4. The anthropophagic id

Due to the dissent and the radicalization of the world around them, Oswald's group, with the adherence of the painter Tarsila do Amaral[7] (1886–1973), 'poked a finger' (Machado, 1928, p. 1) 'at the dumb elites' in the affirmation of the native primitivism of *Abaporu* [man who eats people], created in a telegraphic, contradictory and 'pre-logical'[8] style (Andrade, 1928/1975, p. 1).

The intention of the movement was to confront the many-headed enemy: the 'devouring' sought, in one fell swoop, the extermination of the colonization of the national identity; the political and colonialist elimination of the Franco-Portuguese-Brazilian aesthetic standard; end of the Catholic morality and good manners. It was, in essence, the denunciation of a patriarchal and colonized society, kow-towing to the foreigner (Nunes, 1978, p. XXV), marked by 'base anthropophagy agglomerated with the sins of catechism' and the 'plague of the so-called cultured and Christianized peoples' (Andrade, 1928/1975, p. 8). It was against it all that Anthropophagy offered itself as psychotherapy:

> Only Anthropophagy unites us. Socially. Economically. Philosophically. [...]. The only law of the world. Masked expression of all individualisms, of all collectivisms. Of all religions. Of all peace treaties. *Tupi, or not tupi – that is the question* (...).[9] (Andrade, 1928/1975, p. 7)

After the diagnosis of the Brazilian reality, in tune with the beat of the 'Pau-Brasil' rhythm, the 'Anthropophagic Manifesto' sought to offer therapy on behalf of a new project to all concerned: 'We want the Caraíba Revolution. Greater than the French Revolution. The unification of all effective revolts to the benefit of mankind' (Andrade, 1928/1975, p. 7). And for this, psychoanalysis presented itself as the most valuable instrument to feed the antropophagic face and enhance the 'Caraíba instinct': 'Let's go back to our prehistory. Bring something from this immense, atavistic background. Search the iconic annals. Sieve through the roots of race, with a psychoanalytic approach' (Bopp, 2012, p. 99).

However, in his descent into the unconscious, Freud paid tribute to the Anthropophagus. In affirming Brazilian pre-historic roots, the poets of the Anthropophagy Movement proposed the existence of a state that would render psychoanalysis unnecessary, since the new society would dispense with the catechist evils and Iberian guilt, freeing Brazilians from the Victorian sexual inhibitions and class differences. In short, what seemed to be the best alternative was to send back to Europe its own 'carrion':

> I do not say that someone should eat such meat. It is something that the kitchen has already rejected; the dog did not want, the crows did not accept, threatening to become vegetarians if they insisted. Also leaving it in the larder feeding the carrion flies is not possible. It is therefore best to put the carrion in a tank of creosol and send it back to Europe. (*Revista de Antropofagia*, N. 1, 1928/1975, p. 2)

Thus, rather than merely interpreting the symptoms of modernity, as Freud would have done, Anthropophagy proposed to go one step further and to rehabilitate primitivism, proposing it as a cultural alternative for constructing our identity as 'children of the sun, mother of the living' (Andrade, 1928/1975)[10], leaving behind the world reported by Freud.

It is nevertheless clear that the Anthropophagy project was not only aesthetic. It also launched the proposal for broader social change (Schwarz, 1983, p. 69), as we shall see in the next section.

5. Towards a cure

Modernism had produced a vigorous critique to neutralize colonialist ills and foster a new cultural identity. In order to achieve this, the *Group of 5* proposed the methodology to isolate what they called *Brazilianness*. From this arose stylized Macunaímas, Anthropophagi, Caraíbas, Abaporus and Tupis, that were to become part of the composite 'character' of 'our people'. This period 'idolized mestizo Brazil' (Andrade, 1978, p. 184) and led to the (re)formulation of the country through aesthetics. To achieve this new era, modernism established some stages. The first was the return to the mother tongue of the Brazilian unconscious: 'Catiti Catiti / Imara Notiá / Notiá Imara / Ipeju', as being 'the surrealist jargon' (Andrade, 1928/1975, p. 9). The glorification of the primitive implied a return to an original form of expression, at the same time mediated by language; an intellectual and aesthetic attitude, a distinctive form of expression just as other artists, such as Picasso, were striving towards.

The next step was toward Marx and Weber (Silva, 2006), to propose the rediscovery of indigenous communism: 'We already had communism'.[11] Oswald (1978) revisits the Freudian 'Totem and Taboo' (1913) linking it to the Marxist reading of the patriarchal reality to propose a matriarchal revolution as capable of annihilating the class division and enabling the restitution of property to the Brazilian collective.

Another revolutionary phase was the internal rupture with Judeo-Christian religions. Returning to the idea that religion alienates (Marx), leads to resignation and compassion (Nietzsche) and is used by those in power for the maintenance of paternal authority and alienation, (Freud), Oswald considered that Messianism had been the cornerstone for the maintenance of patriarchialism (Andrade, 2001, p. 104) and colonialism, keeping the colonized submissive to its 'ready-made' truths imported from Portugal (Silva, 2006, p. 119–137).

The last step towards the liberation of the primitive was to be technical progress, allowing the overcoming of capitalist servility, the overcoming of fear and addictions and the control of technologies (Andrade, 2001, p. 106) to 'carry out on earth the leisure promised by the religions in heaven'. After these steps, the three prophets would be left at the door of the matriarchy: after all, 'what sense would the Oedipus complex have in a matriarchy?' (Andrade, 2001, p.

106). The healing direction of Brazilian society was headed toward Utopia, as the plan suggested:

> The repression that generally produces Catholic hysteria, neuroses and illnesses does not exist in a liberated society except in a small percentage, occasioned by the struggle. And direct respite, becoming direct, repairs everything. (Andrade, O., 1929/1992, p. 56)

6. A final note on anthropophagic readings

One of the analytical strategies that have been reaping the greatest benefits for the historical narrative is the quest to understand how the international dissemination of knowledge depends on the development of local cultural tools to allow it to take root in the countries in which it circulates, through its articulation with strategic demands for that collective group. It is possible then to verify that it is not a question of the importance, perfection or veracity of a scientific system or structure, or even its epistemological basis, that guarantees the transfer of knowledge from one context to another. On the contrary, what guarantees the assimilation of knowledge in a given context is a repertoire of references that this knowledge possesses that is able to adhere to the local social experience. It is in this way of reading that the article presented the appropriation of psychoanalysis as a diagnostic tool and therapeutic instrument for Brazilian modernism.

The methodological tool used articulated the concepts of circulation, appropriation and negotiation of Chartier (1988), with the anthropophagic proposals of 'devouring' knowledge according to the context. It was then possible to analyse this knowledge as a system taken by the avant-garde *Intelligentsia* from the framework provided by Freud's text; but also from the *Weltanschauung* arising from the crisis of the European model of civilization; and the imperatives of local modernization projects, as well as the central problem of Brazil's wavering adherence to the European model of civilization.

Notes

1. Juliano Moreira (1873–1933) graduated from Bahia's School of Medicine, where he subsequently worked. Between 1903 and 1930, he headed the National Asylum (in Rio) and was also the Director of the Health Care for the Alienated Asylum. In 1928, he founded Brazilian Psychoanalytical Society – Rio de Janeiro chapter (Facchinetti & Castro, 2015a, p. 18).
2. Fernando Pessoa (1888–1935) was a Portuguese writer and one of the most significant literary figures in the Portuguese language.
3. Formed by Anita Malfatti, Tarsila do Amaral (painters), Menotti del Picchia, Oswald de Andrade and Mário de Andrade (writers), the *Group of Five* was responsible for the ideological and aesthetic references of the Modern Art Week, held at the Municipal Theater of São Paulo, which was a landmark event in Brazilian modernism.

4. Oswald de Andrade (1890–1954) was a Brazilian writer and one of the most controversial personalities of modernism.
5. The Minas Gerais separatist conspiracy (1789) was a movement to liberate Brazil from Portuguese rule.
6. Mario de Andrade (1893–1945) was a Brazilian poet, writer, literary critic, musicologist, folklorist and essayist.
7. Tarsila do Amaral (1886–1973) was a Brazilian painter and one of the central figures in the first phase of the modernist movement in Brazil, alongside Anita Malfatti. Her painting *Abaporu*, of 1928, inaugurates the anthropophagic movement in the plastic arts.
8. Probably an allusion to *La mentalité primitive* (1922), in which Lévy-Bruhl, despite recognizing the existence of a primitive thought, qualifies it as 'pre-logical'.
9. In addition to the obvious parody of Hamlet's quote, the phrase also reflects debates of the period about the first true inhabitants of Piratininga (São Paulo), if they were Tupis, Tapuias or others. On this, see Monteiro (2001).
10. Throughout the 'Manifesto' there are clear allusions to a classic of Brazilian literature of the period: *The Savage*, by Couto de Magalhães (1875/1975), which is often in the sights of the modernists. This part refers to chapter XII of the fifth part, 'Family and wild religion'.
11. Throughout the 'Manifesto' there are clear allusions to a classic of Brazilian literature of the period: *The Savage*, by Couto de Magalhães (1875/1975), as the fifth part of chapter IV, dedicated to the study of 'Communism among the Kayapó'.

Disclosure statement

No potential conflict of interest was reported by the author.

Funding

This work was supported by Conselho Nacional de Desenvolvimento Científico e Tecnológico.

ORCID

Cristiana Facchinetti (iD) http://orcid.org/0000-0003-4879-0307

References

Andrade, M. (1922/1987). *Poesias completes* [The complete poetry]. Belo Horizonte: Itatiaia.

Andrade, M. (1924/1975). Mario's letter to Tarsila. In *Aracy Amaral. Tarsila sua Obra e seu Tempo* [Tarsila, her work, her time] (pp.369–370). São Paulo: Perspectiva/ EDUSP.

Andrade, M. (1928/1993). *Macunaíma, o herói sem nenhum caráter* [Macunaíma, the hero without a character]. Belo Horizonte: Vila Rica.

Andrade, M. (1929/1968). *Mário de Andrade escreve cartas* [The letters of Mário de Andrade]. Rio de Janeiro: Ed. do Autor.

Andrade, M. (1992). Letter excerpt. *Brasilien: Entdeckung und Selbstentdeckung.* Junifestwochen. Zürich: Benteli Verlag.

Andrade, O. (1928/1975). Manifesto Antropófago [Antropophagous manifesto]. In *Revista de Antropofagia. Edição fac-símile.* São Paulo: Abril, Metal Leve S.A.

Andrade, O. (1929/1992). *Estética e Política, ensaios e crítica* [Aesthetics and politics, essays and criticism]. São Paulo: Globo.

Andrade, O. (1978). *Do Pau-Brasil à Antropofagia e às Utopias* [From Pau-Brasil to anthropophagy and utopias]. Rio de Janeiro: Civilização Brasileira.

Andrade, O. (1991). *Ponta de lança* [Spearhead]. São Paulo: Globo.

Andrade, O. (2001). *A utopia antropofágica* [The anthropophagic utopia]. São Paulo: Globo.

Antelo, R. (1986). *Na ilha de Marapatá: Mário de Andrade lê os hispano- americanos* [On the island of Marapatá: Mário de Andrade reads the Hispano-Americans]. São Paulo: HUCITEC.

Bernd, Z. (1992). *Literatura e identidade nacional* [Literature and national identity]. Porto Alegre: Ed. da Universidade.

Birman, J. (2000). A psicanálise e a crítica da modernidade [Psychoanalysis and the critique of modernity]. In Regina Herzog (org.), *A psicanálise e o pensamento moderno.* Rio de Janeiro: Contra Capa Livraria.

Birman, J. (2009). Tradição, memória e arquivo da brasilidade [Tradition, memory and the archive of *Brazilianness*]. *História, Ciências, Saúde - Manguinhos, 16*(1), 195–216.

Boaventura, M. E. (1995). *O salão e a selva: Uma biografia ilustrada de Oswald de Andrade* [The hall and the jungle: An illustrated biography of Oswald de Andrade]. São Paulo: Unicamp.

Bopp, R. (2012). *Movimentos Modernistas no Brasil* [Modernist movements in Brazil]. Rio de Janeiro: José Olympio.

Bradbury, M., & McFarlane, J. (1989). *Modernismo: Guia geral* [Modernism: General guide]. São Paulo: Ed. Cia. Das Letras.

Chartier, R. (1988). *Au bord de la falaise. L'histoire entre certitudes et inquietude* [On the edge of the cliff: History, language and practices]. Paris: Albin Michel.

Facchinetti, C. (2003). Psicanálise modernista no Brasil [Modernist psychoanalysis in Brazil]. *Physis: Revista de Saúde Coletiva, 13*(1), 115–137.

Facchinetti, C. (2012). Psicanálise para Brasileiros [Psychoanalysis for Brazilians]. *Culturas Psi, (1),* 45–62.

Facchinetti, C., & Castro, R.D. (2015a). Die Psychoanalyse als psychiatrisches Werkzeug [Psychoanalysis as a psychiatric tool]. In C. Santos-Stubbe, P. Theiss-Abendroth, & H. Stubbe (Orgs.), *Psychoanalyse in Brasilien: Historische und aktuelle Erkundungen* (pp. 85–112). Gießen: Psychosozial-Verlag.

Facchinetti, C., & Castro, R. D. (2015b). The historiography of psychoanalysis in Brazil. *Dynamis (Granada), 35,* 13–34.

Freud, S. (1915a/2009). Writings on War and Death. *Textos Clássicos de Filosofia*. Coxilhã: Universidade da Beira Interior.

Freud, S. (1915b/1986). Letter to Frederik Van Eeden Vol. XIV. ESB. Rio de Janeiro: Imago.

Freud, S. (1933/1986). Letter from Albert Einstein to Sigmund Freud on July 30, 1932. Vol. XXII. ESB. Rio de Janeiro: Imago.

Hobsbawm, E. (1995). *A era dos extremos: O breve século XX - 1914–1991* [The era of extremes: the brief twentieth century]. São Paulo: Companhia das Letras.

Lander, E. (2005). Ciências sociais: Saberes coloniais e eurocêntricos [Social sciences: colonial and eurocentric knowledge]. In *A colonialidade do saber: Eurocentrismo e ciências sociais - perspectivas latino-americanas* (pp. 21–53). Buenos Aires: Clacso.

Laplantine, F. (2000). *Aprender Antropologia* [Learning anthropology]. São Paulo: Brasiliense.

Machado, A.A. (1928). Abre Alas. *Revista de Antropofagia, I* (1), 1, maio de 1928.

Magalhães. (1875/1975). J.V.C. *O Selvagem* [The Savage]. São Paulo/Belo Horizonte: Edusp/ Itatiaia.

Martins, C.M. (2006, January–June). As metamorfoses em Macunaíma: (Re)formulação da identidade nacional [Metamorphoses in Macunaíma: (re) formulation of national identity]. *Revista eletrônica de crítica e teoria de literaturas, 2* (01).

Mata, L.C. (2013). *Genealogia e primitivismo no modernismo brasileiro* [Genealogy and primitivism in Brazilian modernism] (Doctoral thesis). Florianópolis: UFSC.

Monteiro, J.M. (2001). *Tupis, Tapuias e historiadores* [Tupis, Tapuias and historians]. Campinas, Unicamp.

Moraes, E. J. (2004). As tradições da diversidade cultural – o modernismo [The traditions of cultural diversity – Modernism]. *Seminário Diversidade Cultural Brasileira*. Rio de Janeiro: Casa de Rui Barbosa.

Nunes, B. (1978). Antropofagia ao alcance de todos [Anthropophagy for all]. In: Andrade, Oswald de. *Do Pau-Brasil à Antropofagia e às Utopias* (pp. XI–LII). Rio de Janeiro: Civilização Brasileira.

Pessoa, F. (1998). *Obras em prosa* [Works in prose]. Rio de Janeiro: Nova Aguilar.

Prado, P. (1924/1990). Poesia Pau-Brasil [Pau-Brasil poetry]. In: ANDRADE, Oswald. *Pau-Brasil* (2nd ed). São Paulo: Globo.

Revista de Antropofagia (1928/1975). *Jose Mindlin's facsimile reprint of the first and second dentitions*. São Paulo: Abril/Metal Leve.

Rhodes, C. (1994). *Primitivism in modern art*. London: Thames & Hudson.

Ricoeur, P. (1988). *O Conflito das Interpretações. Ensaios de Hermenêutica* [The conflict of interpretations. Hermeneutics essays]. Rio de Janeiro: Imago.

Russo, J. A. (2002). *O mundo psi no Brasil* [The psy world in Brazil]. Rio de Janeiro: Jorge Zahar.

Sallas, A. L. F. (2010). Narrativas e imagens dos viajantes alemães no Brasil do século XIX [Narratives and images of German travelers in nineteenth-century Brazil]. *História, Ciências, Saúde-Manguinhos, 17*(2), 415–435 [cited 2015-04-03].

Santiago, S. (2000). *Uma literatura nos trópicos* [A literature in the tropics]. Rio de Janeiro: Rocco.

Schwarz, R. (1983). *Que horas são?* [What time is it?]. São Paulo: Companhia das Letras.

Silva, A. P. (2006). *Mário & Oswald: Uma história privada do modernism* [A private history of modernism]. Rio de Janeiro: PUC, Departamento de Letras.

Buddhism, Christianity, and psychotherapy: A three-way conversation in the mid-twentieth century

Christopher Harding

ABSTRACT
This article explores the scope of 'religion-psy dialogue' in the mid-twentieth century, via a case study from Japan: Kosawa Heisaku, a Buddhist psychoanalyst based in Tokyo. By putting this case study in brief comparative perspective, with the conversation that took place in 1965 between Paul Tillich and Carl Rogers, the article discusses both the promise and the pitfalls of the modern and contemporary world of 'religion-psy dialogue', alongside the means by which specialists in a variety of fields might investigate and hold it to account.

BUDISMO, CRISTIANDAD Y PSICOTERAPIA: una conversación en tres direcciones a mediados del siglo

Este artículo explora el alcance del diálogo psicoterapia – religión a mediados del siglo XX, vía el estudio de un caso clinico en Japón: KOSAWA HEISAKU, un psicoanalista budista basado en Tokio. Colocando este estudio de caso en una perspectiva breve, durante una conversación que tuvo lugar en 1965 entre Paul Tillich y Carl Rogers, el artículo presenta dos aspectos: la promesa y los errores del mundo moderno contemporáneo del "diálogo psicoanálisis – religión", así como también los medios por los cuales los especialistas en diferentes campos podrían investigar y llamar a juicio los resultados.

Buddismo, cristianesimo e psicoterapia: una conversazione a tre a metà del XX secolo

Questo articolo esplora la portata del "dialogo religione-psi" a metà del XX secolo, attraverso un caso proveniente dal Giappone: Kosawa Heisaku, uno psicoanalista buddista di Tokyo. Comparando questa esperienza con la conversazione che ebbe luogo nel 1965 tra Paul Tillich e Carl Rogers, l'articolo discute sia le opportunità che le insidie presenti nel "dialogo religione-psi" che caratterizza il mondo moderno e contemporaneo, oltre che i mezzi che potrebbero essere utilizzati da una varietà di specialisti in campi diversi per ampliare tale dialogo.

Bouddhisme, Christianisme et Psychothérapie: une conversation à trois voix au milieu du20ième siècle

Cet article explore le cadre du « dialogue religion-psy » du milieu du 20ième siècle à travers une étude de cas japonaise du psychanalyste bouddhiste Kosawa Heisaku de Tokyo. En comparant cette brève étude de cas avec la conversation qui eut lieu en 1965 entre Paul Tillich et Carl Rogers, l'article discute à la fois la promesse mais aussi les écueils du monde moderne et contemporain du « dialogue religion-psy » ainsi que les moyens par lesquels des spécialistes venant de champs divers pourraient l'examiner et le tenir pour responsable.

Βουδισμός, Χριστιανισμός, και Ψυχοθεραπεία: συζήτηση στα μέσα του 20ου αιώνα

ΠΕΡΙΛΗΨΗ
Το παρόν άρθρο εξετάζει το πεδίο δράσης του «διαλόγου ανάμεσα στη θρησκεία και την ψυχολογία» στα μέσα του 20ουαιώνα μέσα από μια μελέτη περίπτωσης στην Ιαπωνία: Kosawa Heisaku, ένας βουδιστής ψυχαναλυτής στο Τόκυο. Τοποθετώντας αυτή τη μελέτη περίπτωσης σε μια σύντομη συγκριτική οπτική με τη συζήτηση που έλαβε χώρα το 1965 ανάμεσα στον Paul Tillich και στονCarl Rogers, το άρθρο συζητά τόσο τις προοπτικές που ανοίγει όσο και τις παγίδες του μοντέρνου, σύγχρονου κόσμου του «διαλόγου ανάμεσα στη θρησκεία και στην ψυχολογία», παράλληλα με τα μέσα με τα οποία οι ειδικοί από διάφορα πεδία μπορούν να τον διερευνήσουν και να τον αμφισβητήσουν.

What do I do with my distress? This dilemma and its consequences are deeply familiar to psychotherapy. They are also somewhere near the heart of many forms of religious experience. Who am 'I' in the first place? Where in my past, in my relationships, in my habits of behaviour, in my character, should I look for the cause of this distress or for my inability to solve it by myself? Who is this distress turning me into? And is this distress 'mine' alone? Or is it also a judgement against my society, or my conditions of work – perhaps the whole culture that surrounds me?

The evolution of what Nikolas Rose calls the psy disciplines – primarily psychiatry, psychology and psychotherapy – across the twentieth century incorporated a steady shift towards these sorts of wide-ranging, multi-causal approaches to distress, notably though not exclusively in post-Freudian psychoanalytic, Jungian, Existential and person-centred movements. A similar shift occurred, though for different reasons, within religious traditions like Buddhism – both in Asia and in the West – and Christianity: a fresh willingness to extend religious notions of suffering into the medical and the everyday, and to interpret 'healing' more broadly: to include, for example, recovery from, or the religious contextualization of mental illness, addiction and family breakdown. And so we see now books and talks and celebrity figures from the worlds of Buddhism and Christianity making liberal use of psychological terminology, theorizing and case studies. We find pastoral counselling provided across a range of religious traditions, by religious professionals or – increasingly – people with a dual professionalism spanning religion and psychotherapy or counselling. And we encounter the championing of broad benefits for mindfulness meditation, ranging across the personal and inter-relational, the cardiac and neurological, and finally the spiritual and the ethical.

No-one familiar with the introspective, highly psychological writings of the Christian theologian Augustine of Hippo, or the 'moral therapy' precursors to scientific psychiatry could argue that dialogue between the religious and the 'psy' is somehow uniquely a modern phenomenon. And yet it is in the modern era that we find traditions, individuals, institutions, theories, and practices labelled as 'religious' or 'psy' being brought quite self-consciously into contact with counterparts across very real (and generally rather recent) professional and hermeneutic divides.

These points of contact, and the social-historical forces that foster them, matter greatly in the present day because of the broad range of ways in which they are capable of influencing everyday life. Since the 1960s, sociologists and social critics like Philip Rieff and Christopher Lasch, followed more recently by Nikolas Rose and Jan De Vos, have worried about the increasingly pervasive political and cultural power of the psy disciplines. Rose has been particularly concerned about a late twentieth-century trend away from traditional, external modes of surveillance and coercion towards more internalized forms, which feel as though they have been freely chosen by us for our own good:

> Through self-inspection, self-problematization, self-monitoring and confession, we evaluate ourselves according to the criteria provided for us by others. Through self-reformation, therapy, and the calculated reshaping of speech and emotion, we adjust ourselves by means of the techniques propounded by experts of the soul. (Rose, 1999, p. 11)

To then add religion or spirituality into the mix both complicates matters and raises the stakes. Here, are two powerful but rather malleable sources of epistemic and moral authority – religious obligation or faith, and psychological health or well-being – coming together, and capable of producing ideas and practices and ways of being in the world that may hold enormous sway over people while all but defying objective critique. Encompassing in conceptual scope, deeply personal and complex in its everyday reality – ideas, images, and propositions blending with symbol, myth, emotion, faith, presumed unconscious content, and meditative states – religion-psy dialogue seems to resist adequate description, critique and evaluation via any single meta-language.

No surprise, then, that beyond various assertions of their close compatibility – selflessness as morally desirable *and* psychologically beneficial; important analogies across intrapersonal, interpersonal and transpersonal forms of relating (Schreurs, 2006) – lurk complications, antagonisms (albeit sometimes creative ones), points of confusion, and risks to the safety of patients, clients and parishioners. One could extend these concerns, some of which will be explored shortly, even to instances of cultic manipulation and the partial abdication of government responsibility in providing mental healthcare – on the basis, for example, that for some people meditation or membership of a supportive (religious) community may well be sufficient to address their distress.

If these are all good arguments for seeking to unpick the terms and outcomes of religion-psy dialogue, the question arises of how we ought to do it. The variety and complexity involved prohibits any overarching account, although work in this area has tackled various dimensions of dialogue: the alleged corruption of religion by therapeutic as well as late capitalist forces (Carrette & King, 2004), the broad possibilities where 'healing' is concerned (Watts, 2011), and the interface between psychiatry, religion and spirituality (Cook, 2013). In addition to this, by pursuing specific case studies, and then comparing two or more of them, we may find that useful themes and insights emerge: concerning the way in which pioneering thinkers and practitioners exercise power in their work, the nature of the risks to clients that arise as a result, the ways in which clients respond, and the impact upon wider society when hybrid religion-psy ideas make there way out of the consulting room and into wider society (in the form, for example, of everything from professional religious and psychotherapeutic publications to self-help advice for the general reader).

Elsewhere, I have sought to provide a sample framework for how case studies may be carried out and compared (Harding, 2016). In this present article, my aim is to introduce a case-study from mid twentieth-century Japan, and then to suggest the benefits of comparison by showing briefly how some of the themes that arose in Japan find distinct parallels in the United States around the same time.

This comparative or networked (where there are many more than just two) case study approach has the advantage of being less likely to miss the specific historical, cultural and personal dynamics of each instance of dialogue, reminding us that beyond this rather abstract term – 'religion-psy dialogue' – lies no concrete reality, but rather a series of discrete realities, which nevertheless also possess important and informative overlapping features.

Kosawa Heisaku: Buddhism and Psychotherapy

> The smash of the plate reverberates around the kitchen. In the silence that follows the little boy looks up to see his father's fury building. Then out it comes, torrents of recrimination: Why did he do that to a precious plate? Why the hell can this boy never concentrate?
>
> The boy apologizes, means it, but on and on it goes with his father's anger, until the boy can't help but shout back: It was a mistake! And I've tried to apologize! What more do you want?!
>
> But the boy's mother, too, is in the room: People are people, my love, and though what you did was truly wrong, never forget that I know you. And I know you can't help it with things like this – no matter how hard you try.
>
> A sigh escapes the boy's mouth, his shoulders drop. He dissolves into tears: Thankyou mother. Thankyou … I really am sorry. I won't do it again.

A young Kosawa Heisaku offered this 'parable', as he called it, to his readers in the mid-1930s as a way of helping them to appreciate the difference between two sorts of human guilt (Kosawa, 1931). The father gives rise in the boy to the first sort: guilt rooted in fear of punishment, fuelled and warped by enormous hostility. The mother inspires the second: a guilt that Kosawa preferred to call true, revolutionary 'repentance', using a Buddhist term – *zange* – that was to take on enormous significance in Kosawa's personal and professional lives.

Kosawa was a psychiatrist, and one of Japan's first psychoanalysts. He was sure that Sigmund Freud had misunderstood both guilt and religion. A religious state of mind, suggested Freud twenty years before in *Totem and Taboo*, is rooted in an attempt to allay guilt over mankind's primeval slaying of a hated and feared father figure: a long-ago drama that replays itself in the developing psychic lives of young children. But for Kosawa this was not the only – nor the truest – 'religious state of mind'. For that, one has to look at what the mother generates in the boy, as he stands there surrounded by bits of broken plate, his father fuming a few feet away. *I know you. And I know you can't help it with things like this*. To become deeply aware of one's real failings, and then to feel completely met there, known and held by something much greater. Where these twin processes occur, thought Kosawa – whose insights here somewhat parallel those of object relations theorists, Melanie Klein and Donald Winnicott in particular (Ross, 2010) – one finds a liberated state of mind or heart that really does deserve to be called 'religious'.

The parable may well have had origins in the Kosawa family home. Heisaku was born the ninth of ten children, in a village in Kanagawa prefecture where his family owned rice fields. His father, Takatarō – 'hawk-boy' – ran a small bank and dealt in tobacco on the side (Takeda, 1990). Beyond those fields lay Ōyama mountain – known as Aburi-san, or Rainy Mountain, for the heavy dark clouds that regularly burst overhead. Ōyama was a recurring theme in Heisaku's dreams and free associations: he recalled being struck afresh by its beauty on a trip home after long months away; once he remembered – or perhaps imagined – sitting in a mountainside teahouse festooned with wisteria, opening a Viennese umbrella as the rain began to fall (Kosawa, *Furoido sensei kenkyū nōto; yume bunseki*).

Growing up, father and son had relatively little to do with one another. Nine siblings were formidable competition, and the eldest – a girl – was already twenty years old when Heisaku came along, by which time fatherhood for Takatarō may have lost much of its charm. To make matters worse, under Japan's *ie* (household) system, the first son mattered by far the most in terms of family name and inheritance. Heisaku's existence was, at least in this social sense, neither here nor there. His eldest brother's name – 宗栄: Sōei – meant religious glory or honour. Heisaku – 平作 – meant 'normal crop'.

Other than Kosawa's early wish to become Prime Minister, which he attributed to the influence of his father's politics, there is little evidence that Takatarō attended to or shaped the young boy directly in any meaningful way. Kosawa later recalled Takatarō reserving most of his attention instead for the third son of the family, Saburō, who appears to have suffered with behavioural problems. Kosawa resolved to become a psychiatrist one day partly so that he could better understand people like Saburō – how they came to be the way they were, and what might be done about it.

Takatarō's influence on Kosawa was largely indirect, but formidable nonetheless. He plainly scared his son, who found him overbearing, unpredictable, stubborn and fundamentally selfish (Kosawa, *yume bunseki*). He recalled his father once complaining to him about the cost of Heisaku's lengthy hospital treatment for a detached retina while in his mid-20s. Despite this being a serious condition, and doubtless a frightening experience, the only fatherly comments that stayed with Kosawa were that one family member shouldn't be allowed (financially) to destroy the rest. Even as Takatarō lay dying, there was no let up. Kosawa was by this point a fully qualified medical doctor, pursuing a specialism at one of the country's most prestigious universities. His father simply asked him how long he intended to keep messing around 'at school' (Kosawa, *Satogaeri no ki*). Kosawa, for his part, tried to bring what he could of his medical know-how to prolonging his father's life. He was unsuccessful, and may even have blamed himself for his father's early death in 1931.

Two things now happened. First, Kosawa started to identify himself with Prince Ajase, who in a famous Buddhist legend set during the lifetime of the historical Buddha imprisons and then kills his father, King Bimbisara. By the summer of 1931, Kosawa had published a mixed psychoanalytic and religious theory of guilt based on this legend, including in it his parable of the smashed plate. Second, Kosawa left Japan in late 1931 to seek out Sigmund Freud. He wrote to his brother Ichirō – the fourth son, who having inherited the family's money agreed to help finance Kosawa's trip – that his aim was to get Freud's approval for his new 'Ajase Complex' idea and then return to lay his completed thesis at their father's grave (Kosawa, 1932).

In Kosawa's parable, the child's mother appears by contrast as a saintly figure: capable of great patience and gentleness but also possessing a spiritual gift of sorts, able to see into the depths of the child, meet him there, and nurture a 'truly religious state of mind'. Kosawa's own mother, Kon, was a rather more complex figure, and in any case as was common for a family of the Kosawas' standing, the young Heisaku was mostly looked after as a child not by his mother but by a local girl serving as his nanny. 'Ichi' was around ten years old when she began looking after Heisaku, and as one might expect from someone of that age was not entirely committed to the idea of responsible childcare. Missing her friends, she once tied Heisaku to a tree so that he couldn't wander off while she went out to play. Much later in life, Kosawa's thoughts used to return frequently to that moment – a sign, thought one of his students, that his idealization of the maternal possessed deep roots not in satisfaction but in longing and loss (Takeda, 1990).[1]

Kosawa was by no means out of the ordinary here. He grew up in a society many of whose men rhapsodized rather than really knew their mothers (Napier, 1996), and who sought to fix the womanly and the maternal as comforting social, emotional and even spiritual categories. She was, nevertheless, a strong presence in his life, ensuring that 'home' offered a reassuring resonance and embrace for Heisaku – powerful enough to surface years later in his free associations. He remembered her joy when he used to return home from boarding at his Higher School in Sendai, in the north of Japan. Mother would make *amazake* – a sweet rice drink – to welcome him back. She would smile at him as he licked his cup – 'like a baby', he wrote, 'just moving onto solid food'. Heisaku remembered too the vivid sensation of being in the bath with her (Kosawa, *yume bunseki*).

Kosawa's early relationships with his father and mother seem to have shaped his attitudes towards both Buddhism and mental health, and to have inspired his interest in seeing the two placed together in a single, salvific system – albeit with Buddhism and psychoanalysis still retaining separate goals and languages and institutions of their own. Helping to set this emerging conversation in train was a Buddhist monk of the Jōdo Shinshū (Shin) sect by the name of Chikazumi Jōkan. Kosawa met Chikazumi while he was at Higher School in northern Japan, encountering via him a highly devotional, emotional form of Buddhism in which intra-familial relationships were understood as furnishing the individual with transpersonal salvific opportunity. Chikazumi came to this realization while lying in bed one day, critically ill, and hearing his father by his bedside quietly wishing his son's troubles upon himself. It became a moment of conversion: an encounter with compassion so strong and pure that all at once it broke him out of the small, citadel mentality of a young university intellectual, showing him instead a truer, more vital vision of himself – as weak, vulnerable and loved (Iwata, 2011).

The proximate source of this love and compassion was his father. Their ultimate source, for human beings, was the quasi-monotheistic figure of the cosmic Buddha 'Amida' – the Buddha of Infinite Light. The thirteenth-century founder of Shin Buddhism, a man by the name of Shinran, had insisted that the limits of human nature and the boundless compassion of Amida were such that a person needed only to recite a short prayer – *Namu-Amida-Butsu*: 'Hail to Amida Buddha' – in order to be saved. This wasn't some magical formula. Rather, it was an honest and profoundly generative recognition of weakness, such that the very term 'weakness' lost its typical, negative connotations.

Shinran went as far as to say that this prayer could only be truly spoken by Amida Buddha himself, working at the deepest level of a person's subjectivity. As Kai Wariko, a modern Shin poet, put it:

The voice with which I call Amida Buddha

Is the voice with which Amida Buddha calls to me.

For Chikazumi, and soon for Kosawa, the full force of his home life coming into play alongside a new-found devotionalism, modern Japanese family relationships were the means by which Amida's mercy broke into mundane, linear time, and into mundane, human lives (Iwata, 2011).

To twenty-first century ears, much of this must already sound like psychotherapy of a sort (Ross, 2010). But for Kosawa, the connection only really came when he encountered the writings of Sigmund Freud while at university. He found in Freud a modern-day Shinran: someone who understood human frailty, and appeared to be on a quest to tease out and treat them, bringing all the tools of modern science to the task.

A few months spent in Vienna, with Freud and his circle, failed to change Kosawa's mind about Freud and the purpose of psychoanalysis, although he did write home to his brother to say that he was a little disappointed with the general level of psychoanalytic practice in Vienna – and was looking forward to getting home to start his own clinic in Tokyo (Harding, 2014).[2] This he accomplished in 1933, seeing hundreds of clients from all walks of life over the next few years – students, farmers, civil servants, company employees, even a sushi chef, a politician, and a Buddhist monk. From his client records, and from the testimony of those still alive who were treated by Kosawa, we get a sense of the therapeutic fruits of Kosawa's inner religion-psy dialogue across his early life.

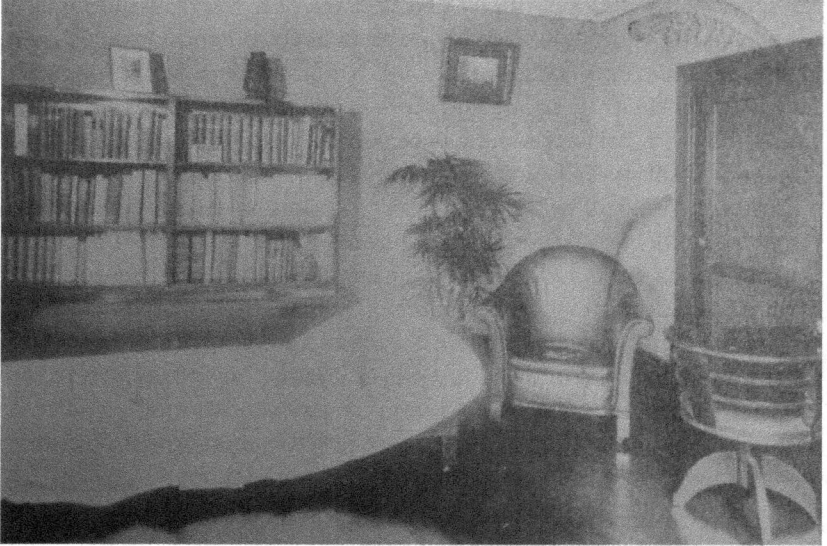

Kosawa's impeccably neutral consulting room – Buddhist conversation with interested clients would instead be held next door, once the session had ended.

Perhaps most revealing are the records of what Kosawa called 'psychoanalysis by mail'. This involved asking clients who couldn't make it for face-to-face sessions in Tokyo to send him, at regular intervals, two documents. The first was a covering letter, addressed to Kosawa. The second was a written record of a period of solo free association – all that had flashed through their heads when they obeyed the standard psychoanalytic command to allow their thoughts and feelings to go where they will. The first document told Kosawa about the client's own self-understanding. The second was the really interesting one: it revealed something of what lurked in the client's unconscious. As therapy went on, Kosawa would hope to see material move from this second document into the first: unconscious elements making their way into conscious awareness.

One client confided in Kosawa that he recalled being embarrassed, as a child, when his parents forced him to wear a girl's rubber swimming cap at the seaside. Kosawa responded that he hadn't been embarrassed at all: he had liked it.

> Covering up the ears symbolizes castration, which in turn suggests your desire to become a girl as a means of securing affection from your father. What's more, your recollection and sharing of that memory now may well be a sign of homosexual feelings towards me …

Perhaps the client spilled his morning tea as he read this. Maybe he glanced nervously over the top of the letter at his father sitting across the table. Whatever happened, this was part analysis, part carefully calibrated attempt to nudge a client who was beginning to over-intellectualize the process of therapy into precisely the kind of gentle, helpless humiliation that Kosawa believed Shinran and Freud were agreed was central to the success of religious practice and psychotherapy alike. One day, a client of Kosawa's reported to him a vivid experience of being momentarily outside of himself, or at least not quite 'in' himself in the usual way. Kosawa was overjoyed. *That*, he said, *is the real aim of psychoanalysis. Without it, psychoanalysis as a technique can never survive* (Harding, 2014).

Religion-Psy Dialogue: Four Emerging Themes

Awareness in the West of the Shin Buddhist sect to which Kosawa belonged has generally been low, despite its considerable size and power in Japan.[3] Buddhism, and especially Japanese Buddhism, has tended to be associated more with Zen. One of the reasons put forward for this is that in Zen, mid-twentieth-century Westerners found a combination they felt Christianity failed any longer to provide: vivid experience, real inner change, minimal theological baggage. Shin Buddhism's emphasis on faith and fundamental human inadequacy, by contrast, was too close for comfort to Protestant, particularly Calvinist Christianity. Why travel thousands of miles to a brand new culture – whether literally or in one's reading – only to find the very thing you were trying to escape?

And yet for all the past and on-going interest in how Zen and psychoanalysis might work together, pioneered in the late 1950s and early 1960s by Erich Fromm and Japan's famous Buddhist evangelist D.T. Suzuki (Fromm, Suzuki, & De Martino, 1960), Shin Buddhism and psychotherapy – as Kosawa's experience shows – possess promising commonalities. So it is all the more interesting to see that just five years after Fromm and Suzuki's work was published, Protestant Christianity and psychotherapy were entering into dialogue via a radio and television studio conversation between the German-American theologian Paul Tillich and Carl Rogers – the latter once having spent time in training for the Christian ministry.

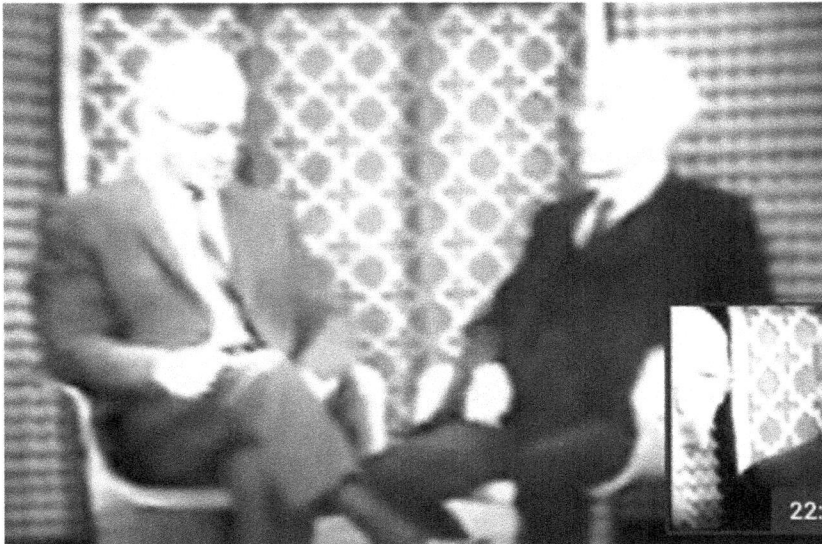

Carl Rogers in conversation with Paul Tillich, filmed for television in 1965.

We may identify four key themes arising in and from Kosawa's inner religion-psy dialogue and the more literal 'dialogue' between Tillich and Rogers: a concern with the damaging social and psychological impact of modernity; a conviction that a profound experience of acceptance lies at the heart of the remedy; a sense that, almost by definition, this cannot be effected by the individual acting alone for his or her own benefit; and a danger – pointed out by critics – that such a remedy, especially where it takes hybrid religion-psy form, risks fostering subjectivities more suited to the totalitarian societies of the recent past in Europe and Japan than their postwar counterparts. It is worth briefly addressing each of these themes in turn.

Kosawa Heisaku was a great critic both of what he saw as pathological individualism in early 1930s Japan and the false community and comfort offered by Marxism and by Japan's 'new religions', the latter striking Kosawa as shallow and manipulative. Kosawa was hardly alone in these concerns: commentators from the novelist Natsume Sōseki through to journalists and philosophers like Watsuji Tetsurō worried about Japan's social and cultural fabric coming apart under the pressure of successive waves of Western fads and fashions from the late nineteenth century onwards. In the United States, both Paul Tillich and Carl Rogers worried, as Terry Cooper has shown (Cooper, 2006), in similar ways. Tillich wrote about 'estrangement': from the ground of our being (a phrase Tillich used frequently for what other theologians called God), from others, and from ourselves. Rogers coined the term 'incongruence': the result of steadily concealing parts of ourselves from others as we grow up, in the hope of making ourselves more acceptable, the end-point of which is the partial concealment of ourselves from ourselves (Cooper, 2006, pp. 17–21).

In all three schemes – Kosawa, Tillich, Rogers – we find that acceptance plays a crucial role in countering all this. Not 'acceptance' in the everyday sense for which 'tolerance' may be the more accurate term, but rather the kind of acceptance that relies on deep knowledge of the person who is being accepted, along with that person's willingness and ability to, as it were, accept the acceptance. One of the reasons why Kosawa chose a little boy, as opposed to an adult, for his parable may be that a little boy, or girl, might still be at the stage where they have not lost their natural ability to accept acceptance. What Rogers called 'conditions of worth', all too clearly communicated in the father's outburst in the parable, have not yet become completely entrenched.

But here is an important point of complication: where does this acceptance come from? For Rogers, the human realm is the source. For Tillich, the human realm – including family and therapist – mediates an acceptance that comes from somewhere well beyond us. Though there are obvious perils in seeking to compare Kosawa's with Tillich's cosmologies, the two share something important in common here. They are convinced that anxiety or other forms of distress stem, in part at least, from our very nature, which in turn is a 'given' of existence rather than something we are capable of shaping. Because of this there is always need of what Tillich called grace and what Kosawa understood as the working of Amida's compassion: some salvific force from without, operating in and through the human.

This places important limits on religion-psy dialogue, in at least two ways. First, though in entirely secular counselling settings one could talk of moments of 'grace' (where something powerful and unintended arises), and on that basis much fruitful conversation can happen between the religion and psy spheres, Tillich's and Kosawa's cosmologies nevertheless understand the human as something else, or more. So for all their usefulness as bridging concepts between the religious and the psy, ideas like 'grace' should not have distinct meanings folded into them as though such things do not matter. Second, in Kosawa's and Tillich's cosmologies human limitations extend to our ability to formulate *any* adequate concepts – suggesting an even more fundamental hermeneutic problem for religion-psy dialogue (Hirota, 2011).[4]

Critics of particular instances of religion-psy dialogue have been quick to offer related cautions. We need some way of distinguishing in meditation, argues one, between psychological insights (about us, in the past and present) and spiritual insights (relating to the 'divine', for wont of a more appropriately inter-religious term, and our place in it, or relationship with it). We need to avoid religion-psy 'dialogue' devolving into the former simply serving the latter – as a provider of high-sounding, inspirational alternative terminologies for what is basically psychology, effectively masking a slide into agnosticism.[5] Still others wonder how forms of Buddhism and Christianity that resist the idea of ultimate reality having a personal dimension can meaningfully talk about 'acceptance'. Surely acceptance is a process with a person at either end (Cooper, 2006; Harding, 2016).

Lastly, there is a concern about what kinds of people some forms of religion-psy dialogue helps to create. Kosawa, in his own day, was accused of literally 'drinking' his clients: thriving on their tales of distress and even playing the saviour to some extent – unable, despite his theorizing to the contrary, to imagine himself rather than Amida Buddha as the source of a person's felt acceptance. An American critic, though not especially well informed about Japan, offered the provocative criticism that whereas psychoanalysis in the United States sought to free the individual from the fetters of society, people like Kosawa actively sought to tighten them. If one stands back and seeks to read, at a purely social level, Kosawa's therapy, then reliant as it was on encouraging an individual to really experience their frailty, inadequacy, and deep need of others it might indeed fit such concerns. Read, however, at a religious or philosophical level, there might seem to have rather more going on: on this reading, *everyone* is heir to the very same constitutional weaknesses, so there can – or at least *should* – be no tyranny of 'strong' over 'weak'. In practice, of course, there was the serious risk of a religious reading glossing, even enabling, the harmful effects described in a social reading. Kosawa was criticized on precisely these grounds by some of his young psychoanalytic trainees.

For Kosawa Heisaku, the fruits of religion-psy dialogue emerged in two simple questions: what is insight, and what does it cost? Good questions, which seem likely to remain with us for some time yet. And there is much to welcome, from this point of view, in the increasing interaction between the religion and psy professions, institutions, ideas and practices – even orientations within individuals. Finding ways to hold such interaction to account, by understanding its sources, claims, motivations and possible implications, is an important task, in which a range of academic and non-academic specialisms have roles to play. This article has sought to sketch out a social-historical and transcultural approach, as just one of many potential angles on this complex modern and contemporary phenomenon.

Notes

1. Another of Kosawa's students, Dr Maeda Shigeharu, agrees, suggesting that Kosawa suffered from not receiving as much love from his mother as he needed. Author interview, March 2016.
2. See also Blowers and Yang Hsueh Chi (1997).
3. An important therapeutic exception is Brazier (2007).
4. On some of the complications of this debate, see Hirota (2011).
5. On the difficult relationships across the twentieth century between Christianity and psychotherapy/counselling, see Johnson and Jones (2000).

Disclosure statement

No potential conflict of interest was reported by the author.

Funding

This work was supported by the Japan Society for the Promotion of Science; Wellcome Trust and British Academy.

References

Blowers, G. H., & Yang Hsueh Chi, S. (1997). Freud's deshi: The coming of psychoanalysis to Japan. *Journal of the History of the Behavioral Sciences, 33*(2), 115–126.
Brazier, C. (2007). *The other Buddhism: Amida comes west*. Philadelphia, PA: O Books.
Carrette, J., & King, R. (2004). *Selling spirituality: The silent takeover of religion*. Abingdon: Routledge.

Cook, C. (2013). *Spirituality, theology, and mental health*. London: SCM Press.
Cooper, T. (2006). *Paul Tillich and psychology*. Macon: Mercer University Press.
Fromm, E., Suzuki, D. T., & De Martino, R. (1960). *Zen Buddhism and psychoanalysis*. New York, NY: Harper & Row.
Harding, C. (2014). Japanese psychoanalysis and Buddhism: The making of a relationship. *History of Psychiatry, 25*(2), 154–170.
Harding, C. G. (2016). Religion, psychiatry, and psychotherapy: Exploring the Japanese experience and the possibility of a transnational framework. *East Asian Science, Technology and Society, 10*(2), 161–182.
Hirota, D. (2011). The awareness of the natural world in Shinjin: Shinran's concept of Jinen. *Buddhist-Christian Studies, 31*, 189–200.
Iwata, F. (2011). *Kindaika no naka no dentōshūkyō to seishinundō: Kijunten toshite no Chikazumi Jōkan kenkyū* [Traditional religion and spiritual movements in the context of modernization: Research on Chikazumi Jokan as a point of reference]. Osaka: Osaka Kyōiku University.
Johnson, E., & Jones, S. (2000). *Psychology and Christianity: Four views*. Downers Grove: IVP USA.
Kosawa, H. (1931, June 15). Seishinbunsekigakujō kara mitaru shūkyō [Religion seen from the perspective of psychoanalysis], Gonryō. Reproduced in English as Two kinds of guilt feelings: the Ajase complex. In K. Matsuki (Ed.), *Japanese contributions to psychoanalysis volume 2* (2007) (pp. 3–11). Tokyo: Japan Psychoanalytic Society.
Kosawa, H. (1932, April 15). *Letter to Kosawa Ichirō*. Tokyo: Kosawa Heisaku Private Family Archive.
Napier, S. (1996). *The fantastic in modern Japanese literature*. Abingdon: Routledge.
Rose, N. (1999). *Governing the soul: Shaping of the private self*. London: Free Association Books.
Ross, J. A. (2010). *Sacred psychoanalysis: An interpretation of the emergence and engagement of religion and spirituality in contemporary psychoanalysis* (PhD thesis). University of Birmingham.
Schreurs, A. (2006). Spiritual relationships as an analytical instrument in psychotherapy with religious patients. *Philosophy, Psychiatry & Psychology, 13*(3), 185–196.
Takeda, M. (1990). *Seishin bunseki to bukkyō* [Psychoanalysis and Buddhism]. Tokyo: Shinchosha.
Watts, F. (Ed.). (2011). *Spiritual healing: Scientific and religious perspectives*. Cambridge: Cambridge University Press.

Inferiority and bereavement: Implicit psychological commitments in the cultural history of Scottish psychotherapy

Gavin Miller

ABSTRACT

The author has argued that psychoanalytic psychotherapy was seen in Scotland as a way to purify Christianity of supernaturalism and moralism, and to propel the faith in a scientifically rational and socially progressive direction. In making this historiographic claim, certain disciplinary protocols are followed, such as the symmetry postulate and a deprecation of reductive psychohistorical explanation. Nonetheless, the contemporary historian of psychotherapy is a psychologized subject whose historical practice rests upon a complex, prereflective background of psychological presuppositions.

INFERIORIDAD Y DUELO: compromisos implícitos en la historia cultural de la Psicoterapia en Escocia- Miller

El autor argumenta que la psicoterapia psicoanalítica en Escocia ha sido vista como una manera de purificar la cristiandad de supernaturalismo y moralidad y propulsar la fe en una dirección cintíficament racional y socialmente progresiva. Al hacer esta afirmación historiográfica, se siguen ciertos patrones disciplinarios, tales como el postulado de simetría y una desaprobación de una explicación psicológica histórica deductiva. Sin embargo, el historiador contemporáneo de la psicoterapia es un sujeto psicologizado cuya práctica histórica descansa sobre el fondo de complejas pre-reflectivas exposiciones psicológicas.

Inferiorità e lutto: impegni psicologici impliciti nella storia culturale della psicoterapia scozzese - Miller

L'autore sostiene che la psicoterapia psicoanalitica è stata vista in Scozia come un modo per purificare il cristianesimo dal soprannaturalismo e dal moralismo e per far avanzare la fede in una direzione scientificamente razionale e socialmente progressista. A questa affermazione storiografica sono seguiti alcuni protocolli disciplinari, come il postulato di simmetria e il biasimo di spiegazioni psico-storiche riduzioniste. Nondimeno, lo storico contemporaneo che si occupa di psicoterapia è un soggetto psicologizzato, la cui pratica si fonda su un complesso background costituito da un pensiero su presupposti psicologici.

Infériorité et deuil: les engagements psychologiques implicites dans l'histoire culturelle de la psychothérapie écossaise - Miller

L'auteur soutient que la psychothérapie psychanalytique était considérée comme étant un moyen d'expurger le christianisme du surnaturel et du moralisme et de propulser la foi dans une direction scientifique rationnelle et socialement progressive. En avançant cet argument historiographique, nous suivons certains protocoles disciplinaires, tels que le postulat de symétrie et l'autodénigrement de l'explication psycho-historique réductrice. Néanmoins, l'historien contemporain de la psychothérapie est un sujet psychologisé dont la pratique historique repose sur un fond complexe et pré-réflectif de présuppositions psychologiques.

Κατωτερότητα και πένθος: Σιωπηρές πολιτισμικές δεσμεύσεις στην πολιτισμική ιστορία της Σκωτσέζικης ψυχοθεραπείας- Miller

Περίληψη: Ο συγγραφέας υποστηρίζει ότι η ψυχαναλυτική ψυχοθεραπεία στη Σκωτία έχει αντιμετωπιστεί ως ένας τρόπος να απαλλαγεί ο Χριστιανισμός από την υπερφυσικότητα και την ηθικολογία, και να προωθήσει την πίστη προς μια επιστημονικά ορθολογική και κοινωνικά προοδευτική κατεύθυνση. Για την υλοποίηση αυτής της ιστοριογραφικής αξίωσης, ακολουθούνται πρωτόκολλα από συγκεκριμένους τομείς, όπως η αρχή της συμμετρίας και η αποδυνάμωση της αναγωγικής ψυχοϊστορικής εξήγησης. Παρόλα αυτά, ο σύγχρονος ιστορικός της ψυχοθεραπείας αποτελεί ένα ψυχολογικοποιημένο υποκείμενο του οποίου οι ιστορικές πρακτικές στηρίζονται σε ένα πολύπλοκο, προστοχαστικό υπόβαθρο ψυχολογικών παραδοχών.

Introduction

For over a decade, I have been working in various ways on the history of psychiatry, psychoanalysis and psychotherapy, in the Scottish context. My research on this topic was originally motivated by an interest in the recovery of neglected local intellectual traditions. But I subsequently discovered that Scotland was particularly informative as a case study in the adaptation of psychotherapeutic ideas and practices to a distinct cultural and national context. The history of psychotherapy in Scotland shows its theoretical and practical adaptation to a context which was unreceptive to the Freudian debunking of religion, and which chose instead to graft psychotherapy into an ongoing constructive critique of the Christian religion by the human sciences. The stimuli of both this special issue and a recently contracted monograph on the topic have encouraged me to reflect on some of the methodological issues raised by this line of research, particularly the place of psychological and psychotherapeutic ideas in my historical practice.

A brief, introductory summary of my work on Scottish psychotherapy may serve to orient readers. A few years into my research, a definite – and perhaps surprising – hypothesis began to emerge about the meaning of Scottish psychotherapy for its leading practitioners. Psychotherapy was seen as an ally to Christian apologetics – as a way to purify Christianity of supernaturalism and moralism, and to propel the faith in a scientifically rational and socially progressive direction (Miller, 2008). Rather than follow the reductive Freudian critique of religious belief and practice, Scottish practitioners tended to ally psychoanalysis and psychotherapy with the rational reconstruction of Christianity by the human sciences, including textual criticism (Miller, 2009, pp. 5–7), social anthropology (Miller, 2008, pp. 39–42) and existential philosophy (Miller, 2009, pp. 7–14). Psychoanalysis was to purge religion of the inessential accretions identified by Freud, such as wish-fulfilment and comforting regression, leaving the way clear for a psychologically reformed faith that emphasized social relations of love and fellowship. An intellectual alliance was created between the Scottish churches and Scottish psychotherapy (Miller, 2007, 2015). Scottish Christianity thus endured, and transformed itself, by drawing on the alliances that it had built in the twentieth century with psychoanalysis and psychotherapy. Even as Scotland rapidly secularized in the 1960s, psychotherapeutic discourses and practices offered a (perhaps temporary) safe haven for Christian life-narrative patterns. Such psychotherapeutic continuation of so-called 'discursive Christianity' (Brown, 2009) appeared in the career of the radical psychiatrist R.D. Laing (Miller, 2009, 2012), as well as in the life and work of less celebrated but nonetheless historically informative exemplars such as the Edinburgh-based psychotherapist Winifred Rushforth (Miller, 2015), and the spiritual-cum-psychotherapeutic milieu that grew up around her (Miller, 2013). Rushforth, for instance, spoke freely and frankly of psychotherapy as a means to miraculous healing and spiritual regeneration (Miller, 2015, pp. 307–310), and such discourses were echoed in Laing's concept of curative *metanoia*, a psychic rebirth that he argued was originally encountered in early Christianity, and represented through metaphors of baptism (Miller, 2009, pp. 14–18).

As a historian, I strive for 'objectivity' by subscribing to well-established disciplinary protocols. In particular, I follow the so-called 'symmetry postulate', by which questions of scientific validity and justification are suspended. This allows me to foreground other explanations for the adoption of psychotherapeutic ideas and practices, including a wide variety of economic, social, cultural and psychological motives and factors. Moreover, I also eschew 'psychohistory', the naïve or reductive historiographic use of psychoanalytic (or psychotherapeutic) explanations that may be favoured by practitioners who pursue the history of their discipline. However, I cannot entirely separate myself from my historical time and place, one in which psychological expertise is widely disseminated and accepted. I may not write from the insider position of a Scottish psychotherapeutic practitioner keen to demonstrate that their particular doctrines emerge by an inner rational necessity. Nonetheless, a broader context of psychological ideas provides the implicit background to my historical practice, offering both fruitful hypotheses and credible explanatory models. The contentious hypothesis of a colonized and 'inferiorist' Scottish intellectual culture has proved heuristically useful to my work, and I have also relied upon the concept of 'discursive bereavement' to explain the translation of Christian discourses into psychotherapeutic form.

Symmetric vs. asymmetric explanation

My research on such cultural factors as religion in the history of Scottish psychotherapy has, in the main, consciously followed the so-called 'symmetry postulate' (also 'symmetry principle'). This long-standing principle in history of science was first established in the sociology of scientific knowledge, and given pre-eminent expression by David Bloor. The symmetry postulate requires that sociology of scientific knowledge should 'be symmetrical in its style of explanation' so that 'the same types of cause' are used to 'explain [...] true and false beliefs' (Bloor, 1991, p. 7). Bloor's important, but elliptical statement gains clarity when contrasted with the asymmetrical style of explanation favoured in earlier histories of science:

> The general structure of these explanations stands out clearly. They all divide behaviours or belief into two types: right and wrong, true or false, rational or irrational. They then invoke sociological or psychological causes to explain the negative side of the division. Such causes explain error, limitation and deviation. The positive side of the evaluative divide is quite different. Here logic, rationality and truth appear to be their own explanation. Here psycho-social causes do not need to be invoked. (Bloor, 1991, p. 9)

The symmetrical style of explanation proper to the sociology of scientific knowledge, however, offers psycho-social causes for both 'right' and 'wrong' beliefs, rather than explaining the former's social currency by their truthfulness, and the latter's by extraneous historical factors.

The symmetry postulate thereby contrasts with what might be called the everyday attitude of scientific agents, including psychotherapeutic researchers and practitioners. As a general rule, we may safely presume that psychotherapists typically hold the theory behind their practice to be valid and justifiable. Obviously, there are caveats to such a rule: practitioners may believe that theory poorly understands practice, or requires refinement or elaboration – and perhaps there is even a minority who have no belief in their method, but practise psychotherapy instead in a spirit of conscious charlatanry. Nonetheless, the typical psychotherapist adheres to the particular doctrine of their approach, be what it may (cognitive-behaviourist, existential-humanist, psychoanalytic, etc.). And, no doubt, those of us who are potential consumers of psychotherapy are ethically reassured by practitioners who believe in what they do.

The reasons for adherence to a particular psychotherapeutic body of theory and practice are surely manifold. But, regardless of the exact reasons in any particular case, the practitioner's trust in the validity of their approach presents a potential obstacle to their historiographical competence. The practitioner's natural inclination is to explain the currency of their ideas by reference to their truth and rational validity. A follower of Fairbairn might argue, for instance, that the Scottish psychoanalyst's theory of the unconscious mind grasps more readily phenomena that evade the Freudian grasp – such as the now widely recognized moral defence, in which the abused or neglected child internalizes its own sinfulness, rather than acknowledge the yet more terrible reality of its parents' badness (Fairbairn, 2002). A Fairbairn-style therapist might then tend to offer asymmetric psycho-social explanations for the currency of rival, 'mistaken' approaches. If we ask her to explain the currency of, say, cognitive-behavioural therapy, our hypothetical practitioner may well make reference to the limited time available in professional practice, the restrictive and biomedically inflected evidentiary models that are promulgated in the health professions and the bureaucratic fondness for therapeutic approaches that are readily translated into generalized protocols. In short, our hypothetical Fairbairn follower will (be inclined to): (a) explain the fact of her belief in Fairbairn's psychoanalytic psychotherapy by its rational validity; (b) explain the fact of belief by others in contradictory schools by reference to a host of economic, social, cultural and psychological motives and factors, such as economic expediency, cultural (including professional) prejudices and organizational functionality.

This asymmetric style is entirely appropriate in the everyday attitude of the psychotherapeutic practitioner, for Bloor's symmetry postulate is a methodological principle rather than an assault upon scientific rationality (Bloor, 1991, pp. 175–179). However, with the aid of the symmetry principle, the historian or sociologist can deliberately neglect, suspend or bracket scientific validity and justification in order to concentrate upon the kinds of explanation where socio-historical reasoning gains purchase. The symmetry postulate is a productive falsification, like such concepts as 'centre of gravity', 'economically rational actor', or the 'the square root of a negative number'. There is no absurdity in simplifying or falsifying an object to know it better. As Hans Vaihinger explains, 'many thought-processes and thought-constructs appear to be to be consciously false assumptions, which either contradict reality or are even contradictory in themselves' (Vaihinger, 1924, pp. xlvi, xlvii). So the historian of psychotherapy may proceed *as if* disciplinary validity has no part to play in the explanation of why certain theories and practices are adopted. Thus, as a historian of Scottish psychotherapy, rather than a practitioner, I explain the fact of belief in psychotherapy by reference to non-rational factors, including economic, cultural, organizational, societal and psychological causes. With regard to the distinctive schools of Scottish psychotherapy, I argue that these causes include: a context of Christianized evolutionary theory and sociology that operated as a philosophical customs point for Freudian ideas; the ethical authority and social ambition of twentieth-century organizational Christianity; and the appeal of preserving Christian discursive patterns, including Christian life narratives (Miller, 2008, 2012, 2014, 2015).

Against (and for) 'psychohistory'

The symmetry principle tends to distance the academic historian of psychotherapy from the practitioner. Even where these roles are combined in a single person, performance of each seems to have quite different requirements. This separation of historian from psychotherapist is intensified by the former's aversion to 'psychohistory', which is regarded by academics as the naïve and reductive historiographic application by practitioners of their favoured psychological (and often psychotherapeutic) concepts. The explanatory ambitions of psychohistory are currently realized by The Association for Psychohistory and the periodical it has produced since 1976, *The Journal of Psychohistory* (http://psychohistory.com/the-journal-of-psychohistory). Readers will find in recent abstracts of the journal a variety of psychologized explanations of historical phenomena. The election of Donald Trump as US President in 2016, for instance, has provoked psychohistorical explanation of the man, his electoral appeal and the consequences of his success, with the invocation of such concepts as narcissism, denial and splitting. Other recent articles show a particular interest in the explanatory power of trauma, both in the individual – particularly in childhood – and in an entire community across generations.

As well as following the symmetry postulate, I have therefore tried to avoid the practitioner categories of psychohistory, particularly with application to Scottish culture. The flexible psychohistorical doctrine of intergenerational trauma does not yet seem to have gained much currency in Scottish historiography. However, other practitioner-led psychohistorical narratives have gained credence in recent years, despite their deficient academic standing. The counsellor and trainer Carol Craig diagnoses the Scots in her manifesto *The Scots' Crisis of Confidence* (2003) using Jungian typologies. In her view, the Scottish nation is psycho-culturally distinguished by a preference for 'thinking judgement' (Craig, 2003, p. 58) and for dwelling in the 'extravert rather than the introvert world' (Craig, 2003, p. 48). The consequence is that the Scots are practical fellows with lively inquiring minds, but are emotionally illiterate and hyper-critical of themselves and others – hence their typically low self-confidence (Craig, 2003, pp. 48, 49, 59). Remarkably, Craig's diagnosis led to the founding of a Centre for

Confidence and Well-Being (2004-present) which received both charitable support and Scottish Executive/Scottish Government funding (http://www.centreforconfidence.co.uk/). The Centre also promoted so-called 'positive psychology', which controversially calls for the disciplined cultivation of positive emotion as a means to greater health, productivity and social cohesion (Ehrenreich, 2009). Latterly, Craig has deprecated positive psychology, instead promoting 'well-being', and drawing upon evolutionary psychology to explain the neoliberal recrudescence of atavistic patterns of primate dominance and submission (Craig, 2010).

The academic response to Craig's psychohistorical diagnosis and therapeutics illustrates why historians distance themselves from such practitioner-led analyses. The anthropologist A.P. Cohen dismisses Craig's account as 'misconceived theory' and a 'concoction of simplistic generalisations': 'She sees Scottish society as generalisable into a collective psyche to which she applies terms drawn from Jungian analysis, and from which she derives a deterministic culture which explains pretty well everything from economic failure to dreary conformity' (Cohen, 2004, p. 160). Yet, as much I have eschewed this particular national diagnosis and its counterparts (e.g. Miller, 2005), I cannot entirely dismiss psychohistorical analysis of Scottish culture. In *The Eclipse of Scottish Culture*, Ronald Turnbull and Craig Beveridge explain that they

> rely on the concept of inferiorisation, which was developed by Frantz Fanon in his account of the psycho-cultural dimension of national subordination in the Third World. Fanon argues that the native comes to internalise the message that local customs are inferior to the culture of the coloniser, a theme which runs through cultural production in the colony. (Beveridge & Turnbull, 1989, p. 1)

Beveridge and Turnbull argue that 'images of backwardness and inferiority [...] govern the Scottish intelligentsia's discourse on Scotland', a rhetoric which can be explained in their view only by 'the loss of self-belief and acceptance of the superiority of metropolitan mores engendered by the sustained and ubiquitous institutional and ideological pressures which are exerted by "core" powers on their satellites' (Beveridge & Turnbull, 1989, p. 112). The colonial status of Scotland is certainly debatable (although perhaps defensible in terms of 'internal colonisation' (Hechter, 1975)), and a rigorous social scientific investigation of Beveridge and Turnbull's thesis would indeed be daunting. Yet, as part of what might loosely be called a 'context of discovery', I have found Beveridge and Turnbull's thesis a useful spur to historical investigation. It has encouraged me to ask what *if* Scottish intellectual life were systematically 'inferiorist' – what might have been overlooked? Beveridge and Turnbull's psycho-cultural reading has thus been useful to me as a heuristic device, notwithstanding the reality of inferiorist attitudes in the Scottish population.

Implicit psychologies in academic history of psychotherapy

I may not wholly subscribe to Fanon's analysis, and its psychological assumptions, in a Scottish context (although it does make remarkable sense of Craig's peculiar worldview, as well as other unusual claims about Scottishness (e.g. Miller, 2004)). However, there are other areas of my work where psychological theses are implicit not merely in the creation of fruitful lines of investigation, but in the historical explanation itself. Steven Sutcliffe, following Callum Brown's historical analysis, refers to the 'striking response to the "discursive bereavement" (the grief at the cultural loss of religious certainties) experienced mid-century by Christians' (Sutcliffe, 2010, p. 195) – including the radical Scottish psychiatrist R.D. Laing (1927–1989). In Brown's history of Christianity, the primary form of Christian religious life is discursive, and upon it institutional and associational forms are dependent: the believer (and often the secularized, former believer) understands him or her self through narrative categories of 'a life-journey, using notions of progression, improvement and personal salvation, whether within religion or opposing it' (Brown, 2009, p. 185). Following Sutcliffe and Brown, I have delineated in my own work a cultural response whereby Scottish psychotherapy took on, and refurbished, such Christian narratives. Laing's autobiography *Wisdom, Madness and Folly* (Laing, 1998), for instance, has an implicitly Christian biographical structure arranged around a series of turning points – this is why, for instance, he encodes his radical disenchantment with conventional psychiatry as a Pauline conversion (Miller, 2012, pp. 141, 142). A similar pattern is also important in the life and work of the far more obscure Scottish psychotherapist, Winifred Rushforth (1885–1983), and in the discourses and practices of the Edinburgh-based Davidson Clinic which she directed. Rushforth and her collaborators self-consciously grafted Christian life-narrative patterns such as rebirth and miraculous healing into psychoanalytic and psychotherapeutic discourse – even to the extent of seeing Providential forces at work in the founding of their organization (Miller, 2015, p. 309).

The work of Brown, and also Sutcliffe, has offered me a way of explaining the investment by some Scottish Christians in psychotherapy, even as postwar secularization intensified: the scientific authority of psychotherapy legitimated their discursive and practical continuation of Christian life-narrative patterns to which they were deeply attached. However, it seems inescapable to me that Brown's concept of a 'discursive bereavement' (Brown, 2009, p. 184) has credibility because it draws upon a variety of implicit psychological positions. Brown's concept of a Christian life-narrative pattern clearly relies upon an implicitly cognitivist psychology. The Christian's life narrative selects and links together particular items of experience into a particular schematic pattern – such constructive activity is familiar from proto-cognitivist work such as Bartlett's famous study of memory (Bartlett, 1995), and from self-consciously 'cognitivist' psychology in the research programme given an identity by Ulrich

Neisser in the 1960s (Neisser, 1967). Nor is this schematic pattern purely cogni-tivist in significance, for it is reflexively internalized in the way theorized by social psychologists in the constructionist school, such as Kenneth Gergen (Gergen, 1973, 1985). Brown thus refers to the 'subjectification' of Christian discourses – not just 'a personal process of subscription to often very public discourses', but also 'very private (indeed sometimes intensely secret) protocols related to those discourses' (Brown, 2009, p. 13). Moreover, Brown's concept of 'discursive bereavement' manifestly identifies feelings of 'loss' experienced by Christian subjects who have witnessed, and undergone, the 'discourse change' of secular-ization (Brown, 2009, p. 184). The language of 'loss' and 'bereavement' implicitly deploys psychologized ideas of grief and mourning which have flourished over the past century or so, and transposes them to the loss of a discourse rather than a person. As Leeat Granek explains, the work of psychological experts such as Freud and Helene Deutsch has made our common sense about grief a highly theorized psychological construct (Granek, 2010, pp. 50–54). Amongst our everyday psychologized assumptions are

> the idea that grief is an active process that involves an intense struggle to give up the emotional attachment to the person who has been lost, and that this struggle is a process that involves time and energy on the part of those mourning. (Granek, 2010, p. 52)

Moreover, it is assumed that 'the death of a loved person must produce a reac-tion in the bereaved, and that the absence of such grief is as much pathology as is extensive mourning in time and intensity' (Granek, 2010, p. 53).

Brown's concept of 'discursive bereavement' implicitly psychologizes Christianity as a social-cognitivist discourse that constructs the believer's experi-ence, which may be reflexively internalized in a socially constructionist manner, and which – if lost – may be the object of loss or grief in the way theorized in psychoanalytic and post-psychoanalytic discourses. This complex syncretism of different concepts from quite varied psychological schools (some of which may be in tension with each other) has been important in my work at an explanatory as well as heuristic level. The concept of 'discursive bereavement', like 'inferio-rism', certainly gives me a sense of interesting phenomena to look out for. But it is more than simply a scaffolding that can be removed once the edifice of argument is complete. Discursive bereavement is also something which I see evidenced in the life and work of Laing, Rushforth and others: the phenomenon seems to me real, and explicable in the ways implied by Brown's concept. This commitment to the reality of discursive bereavement prevents me from repre-senting it merely as a productive methodological fiction. It is not *as if* R.D. Laing were adapting psychotherapeutic materials to Christian discursive patterns in order to deal with the loss of faith that beset him in an era of secularization. That is what he was doing and why. There is, then, no magic chalk circle into which I can retreat: I am, in my historiography of Scottish psychotherapy, implicitly endorsing – via Brown's concept – social cognitivist and social constructionist psychologies, as well as psychoanalytic and post-psychoanalytic accounts of attachment, loss and mourning.

Conclusion

Given that my procedures of discovery and explanation are definitely, albeit implicitly, psychologized, I must sound a note of warning about the category 'psychohistory'. This concept certainly can be used – against the intentions of its practitioners – to demarcate psychologizing explanations that are reductive, overambitious, mono-causal or deprecated in some other way (e.g. by seeming to the historiographer to be implausible or unlikely). But in doing so, one must be careful not to give the impression that psychologized historical explanation is the sole domain of psychotherapeutic practitioners who are invested in the validity of their particular theory and method. A related caution applies to the symmetry postulate, and its distancing of the historian from psychological valid- ity claims: the historian of psychotherapy may proceed *as if* psychothothera- peutic validity has no part to play in the explanation of why certain theories and practices are adopted. However, the historian's own activity will surely invoke 'psycho-social causes' (Bloor, 1991, p. 9) if it aims at adequacy, and thus presume the validity of various psychological school and theses. Valid methodological postulates such as the symmetry principle, and scepticism about practitioner histories, are of great value to cultural history of psychotherapy. However, they should not conceal the extent to which any contemporary researcher, myself included, is caught up always and already in a complex background of psy- chologized presuppositions. The contemporary historian is as psychologized as any other modern subject, including those impertinent practitioners, with their folk histories of psychotherapy. Accordingly, I at least do not know what historiography purged of psychological presuppositions would look like – how else would I explain what Laing or Rushforth were experiencing and doing, except using categories that I in fact hold as valid?

My particular argument here is more generally encapsulated by the historio- graphic recognition, post-Gadamer, that '[w]e are more subject to history than it can be subjected to consciousness. Whenever we understand, history effects the horizon, never susceptible of ultimate clarification, of everything that can appear meaningful and worth inquiring into' (Grondin, 1994, p. 114). My practice of historical reason is itself historically and culturally situated, and so rests upon a background of pre-judgements which include any number of psychological and psychotherapeutic explanatory forms. Objectivity in this process cannot consist of simply suspending my own judgement on psychological validity claims. The symmetry postulate is appropriate for the historical agents under investigation (I do not explain their beliefs by their putative greater rational validity). But I must accept that I am continually selecting, using and evaluating forms of psycho-social explanation that have some affinity to the psychotherapeutic discourses employed by the practitioner community that I investigate. While I oppose historical investigations that are psychologically reductive, or one-sided, or otherwise deficient, I am nonetheless entangled with psychological debates. As a psychologized subject of a psychologized era, I write history of psychotherapy that is implicitly (and at times explicitly) psychological, and which addresses a psychologized audience. My distance from the psychotherapeutic community which I examine can only ever be partial: there is no psychological 'view from nowhere' to which I have access.

Disclosure statement

No potential conflict of interest was reported by the author.

References

Bartlett, F. C. (1995). *Remembering: A study in experimental and social psychology*. Cambridge: Cambridge University Press.

Beveridge, C., & Turnbull, R. (1989). *The eclipse of Scottish culture: Inferiorism and the intellectuals*. Edinburgh: Polygon.

Bloor, D. (1991). *Knowledge and social imagery* (2nd ed.). Chicago, IL: University of Chicago Press.

Brown, C. G. (2009). *The death of Christian Britain: Understanding secularisation 1800–2000* (2nd ed.). London: Routledge.

Cohen, A. P. (2004). Review: Scots' crisis of confidence. *Scottish Affairs, 49*(First Series), 160–162.

Craig, C. (2003). *The Scots' crisis of confidence*. Edinburgh: Big Thinking.

Craig, C. (2010). *The tears that made the Clyde: Well-being in Glasgow*. Glendaruel: Argyll Publishing.

Ehrenreich, B. (2009). *Smile or die: How positive thinking fooled America and the World*. London: Granta.

Fairbairn, W. R. D. (2002). *The repression and the return of bad objects (with special reference to the 'War Neuroses') psychoanalytic studies of the personality* (pp. 59–81). London: Routledge.

Gergen, K. J. (1973). Social psychology as history. *Journal of Personality and Social Psychology, 26*(2), 309–320.

Gergen, K. J. (1985). The social constructionist movement in modern psychology. *American Psychologist, 40*(3), 266–275.

Granek, L. (2010). Grief as pathology: The evolution of grief theory in psychology from Freud to the present. *History of Psychology, 13*(1), 46–73.

Grondin, J. (1994). *Introduction to philosophical hermeneutics*. (J. Weinsheimer, Trans.). New Haven, CT: Yale University Press.

Hechter, M. (1975). *Internal colonialism: The Celtic fringe in British national development, 1536–1966*. London: Routledge and Kegan Paul.

Laing, R. D. (1998). *Wisdom, madness, and folly: The making of a psychiatrist 1927–57*. Edinburgh: Canongate.

Miller, G. (2004). 'Persuade without convincing … represent without reasoning': The inferiorist mythology of the Scots Language. In E. Bell & G. Miller (Eds.), *Scotland in theory: Reflections on literature and culture* (pp. 197–209). New York, NY: Rodopi.

Miller, G. (2005). National confessions: Queer theory meets Scottish literature. *Scottish Studies Review, 6*(2), 60–71.

Miller, G. (2007). John Macmurray's psychotherapeutic Christianity: The influence of Alfred Adler and Fritz Künkel. *Journal of Scottish Thought, 1*(1), 103–121.

Miller, G. (2008). Scottish psychoanalysis: A rational religion. *Journal of the History of the Behavioral Sciences, 44*(1), 38–58.

Miller, G. (2009). R.D. Laing and theology: The influence of Christian existentialism on *The Divided Self*. *History of the Human Sciences, 22*(2), 1–21.

Miller, G. (2012). R.D. Laing's theological hinterland: The contrast between mysticism and communion. *History of Psychiatry, 23*(2), 139–155.

Miller, G. (2013). Resisting self-spirituality: Counselling as spirituality in the dialogues of Hans Schauder and Marcus Lefébure. *Journal of Contemporary Religion, 28*(1), 125–140.

Miller, G. (2014). Making Fairbairn's psychoanalysis thinkable: Henry Drummond's natural laws of the spiritual world. In G. S. Clarke & D. E. Scharff (Eds.), *Fairbairn and the object relations tradition* (pp. 41–48). London: Karnac.

Miller, G. (2015). Winifred Rushforth and the Davidson Clinic for Medical Psychotherapy: A case study in the overlap of psychotherapy, Christianity and New Age spirituality. *History of Psychiatry, 26*(3), 303–317.

Neisser, U. (1967). *Cognitive Psychology*. New York, NY: Appleton-Century-Crofts.

Sutcliffe, S. (2010). After 'The Religion of My Fathers': The quest for composure in the 'Post-Presbyterian' self. In L. Abrams & C. G. Brown (Eds.), *A history of everyday life in twentieth-century Scotland* (pp. 181–205). Edinburgh: Edinburgh University Press.

Vaihinger, H. (1924). *The philosophy of 'as if': A system of the theoretical, practical, and religious fictions of mankind*. (C. K. Ogden, Trans.). London: Routledge.

Towards trans-cultural histories of psychotherapies

Hans Pols

ABSTRACT

Psychotherapy is a regulated form of verbal interaction, which necessarily incorporates broader shared cultural assumptions and narrative templates. Like any form of verbal interaction, it is fluid, adaptable and malleable, particularly when it enters new cultural domains. The increasing global penetration of psychotherapeutic techniques calls for an analysis of the changes, modifications, and innovations of its techniques and accompanying theories. This will eventually allow scholars to view European and North American forms of psychotherapy as variations tied to specific locations and cultures. Tracing the trans-national and trans-cultural dissemination of psychotherapeutic theories and techniques allows historians to chart their inherent variability, test limits, and analyse the broader social and political uses of psychotherapy within different national and cultural contexts. In addition to investigating psychotherapy in its various manifestations, historians should continue to inquire about its personal, social and political uses.

PR2. HACIA UNA HISTORIA TRANSCULTURAL DE LAS PSICOTERAPIAS: Comentario

La psicoterapia es una forma de interacción verbal regulada, la cual necesariamente incorpora amplias suposiciones y esquemas narrativos. Es altamente fluida, adaptable y maleable, en particular cuando entra dentro de ámbitos culturales nuevos. El aumento en la penetración global de las técnicas psicoterapéuticas, requiere del análisis histórico de los cambios, modificacions e innovaciones de sus técnicas y de las teorías que las acompañan. Eventualmente, ésto permitirá a los investigadores, comprender las formas de psicoterapia europea y norteamericana como variaciones ligadas a localizaciones y culturas específicas. Trazar la diseminación trans-nacional y trans-cultural de las teorías y ténicas psicoterapéuticas, permite a los historiadores registrar su inherente variabilidad, probar los límites y analizar la amplitud de los usos políticos y sociales de la psicoterapia dentro de diferentes contextos nacionales y culturales. La psicoterapia puede estimular y desanimar a la vez el compromiso social y politico. Además, al investigar la psicoterapia en sus diferentes manifestaciones, los historiadores deberán continuar indagando acerca de su utilización en los aspectos personales, sociales y politicos.

Verso storie trans-culturali di psicoterapie - Un commento

La psicoterapia è una forma regolata di interazione verbale che incorpora necessariamente ampi presupposti e modelli narrativi culturalmente condivisi. Come ogni forma di integrazione verbale strutturata, è altamente fluida, adattabile e malleabile, in particolare quando incontra ambiti culturali nuovi. La crescente espansione globale delle tecniche psicoterapeutiche necessita di un'analisi storica dei cambiamenti, delle modifiche e delle innovazioni relative alle tecniche e alle teorie. Questo consentirà di considerare le forme di psicoterapia europee e nordamericane come "variazioni" collegate a specifici luoghi e culture. Schematizzare la diffusione transnazionale e transculturale di teorie e tecniche psicoterapeutiche consente agli storici di tracciare la loro variabilità intrinseca, testare i limiti e analizzare i più ampi usi socio-politici della psicoterapia all'interno di diversi contesti nazionali e culturali. La psicoterapia infatti può sia incoraggiare che attenuare l'impegno sociale e politico. Risulta effettivamente importante indagare le varie manifestazioni della psicoterapia, ma anche continuare a documentarne gli usi personali, sociali e politici.

PR 2. Vers des histoires transculturelles des psychothérapies – un commentaire

La psychothérapie est une forme d'interaction verbale régulée incorporant nécessairement des présupposés culturels et des formats narratifs partagés. Comme toute forme d'intégration verbale structurée, elle est hautement fluide, adaptable et malléable, en particulier quand elle entre dans de nouveaux domaines culturels. La pénétration globale de plus en plus importante des techniques psychothérapeutiques demande une analyse historique des changements, modifications et innovations de ses techniques et des théories qui les accompagnent. Ceci permettra éventuellement aux chercheurs de considérer les formes européenne et nord-américaine de psychothérapie comme des variations attachées à des lieux et à des cultures spécifiques. Localiser la dissémination transnationale et transculturelle des théories et des techniques psychothérapeutiques permet aux historiens de rendre compte de leur variabilité inhérente, de tester les limites et d'analyser les utilisations sociales et politiques au sens large de la psychothérapie au sein des différents contextes nationaux et culturels. La psychothérapie peut à la fois promouvoir et freiner l'engagement social et politique. En plus d'investiguer la psychothérapie dans ses manifestations multiples, les historiens devraient continuer à s'interroger sur ses utilisations personnelles, sociales et politiques.

Προς μια διαπολιτισμική ιστορία της ψυχοθεραπείας- Ένα σχόλιο

Η ψυχοθεραπεία αποτελεί μια ελεγχόμενη μορφή λεκτικής αλληλεπίδρασης, η οποία ενσωματώνει ευρύτερες κοινές πολιτισμικές παραδοχές και αφηγηματικά πρότυπα. Όπως κάθε μορφή δομημένης λεκτικής απαρτίωσης, είναι ιδιαίτερα ρευστή, προσαρμόσιμη και εύπλαστη, ιδιαίτερα όταν εισέρχεται σε νέους πολιτισμικούς τομείς. Η παγκοσμίως αυξανόμενη διείσδυση των ψυχοθεραπευτικών τεχνικών απαιτεί μια ιστορική ανάλυση των μεταβολών, των τροποποιήσεων και των καινοτομιών των τεχνικών και των θεωριών που τη συνοδεύουν. Αυτό εντέλει θα επιτρέψει στους μελετητές να αναγνωρίσουν τις ευρωπαϊκές και βορειοαμερικανικές μορφές ψυχοθεραπείας ως παραλλαγές που

συνδέονται με συγκεκριμένες περιοχές και πολιτισμούς. Η μελέτη της διακρατικής και διαπολιτισμικής διάδοσης των ψυχοθεραπευτικών θεωριών και τεχνικών επιτρέπει στους ιστορικούς να καταγράψουν την εγγενή ποικιλομορφία τους, να εξετάσουν τα όρια και να αναλύσουν τις ευρύτερες κοινωνικές και πολιτικές εφαρμογές της ψυχοθεραπείας μέσα σε διαφορετικά εθνικά και πολιτισμικά πλαίσια. Η ψυχοθεραπεία μπορεί να ενθαρρύνει αλλά και να μειώσει την κοινωνική και πολιτική δράση. Πέρα από τη διερεύνηση της ψυχοθεραπείας στις διάφορες εκδηλώσεις της, οι ιστορικοί οφείλουν να συνεχίσουν την έρευνα γύρω από τις προσωπικές, κοινωνικές και πολιτικές χρήσεις της.

Patterns of verbal interaction are, by their nature, adaptable, fluid and malleable. Psychotherapy is a structured form of verbal interaction that takes place in an asymmetric and generally dyadic relationship between two human beings. Because it is an abstracted and regulated form of everyday human interaction, it inevitably incorporates culture-specific narrative styles and templates, framing and plot devices, and story-lines. It is grounded in shared cultural understandings and narrative repertoires, so that specific forms of psychotherapy practised at specific times, locations and cultural settings will have distinct local inflections. Because psychotherapy aims to be an interpretive technique that gives meaning to past experiences and present difficulties that have defied the interpretative abilities of clients, however, practitioners often introduce additional narrative elements that are not always congruent with shared cultural understandings. The ability to construct narratives, giving novel meanings to past or current experiences, gives psychotherapeutic interventions their transformative potency. Psychotherapy both replicates and aims to transcend specific cultural framings of distress, which makes the analysis of its trans-national and trans-cultural transmission unusually interesting.

The techniques used by psychotherapists are flexible and malleable; throughout history they have been appropriated, transformed, updated and re-interpreted in order to make them meaningful in new situations and different cultural settings. As a semi-structured discursive practice necessarily relying on shared cultural codes, it is virtually impossible to make psychotherapy into an immutable mobile (as Latour (1990) would have phrased it), despite the repeated and almost obsessive claims of scientific neutrality. It is similarly impossible to enclose professional boundaries around psychotherapy to make it the exclusive property of a defined group of professionals who claim that they are uniquely qualified to employ them. Despite attempts to standardise and rationalise psychotherapeutic techniques in order to contain its inherent variability and limit the creativity of practitioners, successive and continuing appropriations of its theorisations, rationalisations and techniques have produced numerous original and imaginative iterations.

To transplant psychotherapy to novel locations requires engaging in dialogues with specific cultural narratives. Interestingly, once these dialogues are opened, they have the potential to changes these cultural narratives, as they become psychologised. Psychological approaches to the self, with their accompanying vocabularies, have influenced and altered, to strikingly different degrees, popular understandings of self, the purpose of life, and human nature as well as culturally specific idioms of distress and generally accepted means of articulating personal difficulties. The various ways in which 'psy' transforms local cultural idioms provide interesting areas of study for historians, sociologists and anthropologists. It also is a reminder that it is impossible to study the trans-national dissemination of psychotherapy and the development of local and specific cultures separately; both develop in dynamic interaction.

Many psychotherapists have a keen interest in history (Marks, 2017). Some look for precursors and antecedents as far back in history as they can find them; others go to great lengths to link their specific approach to leading psychotherapists and esteemed psychotherapeutic traditions. Several histories written by psychoanalysts claim that psychotherapy first appeared when Sigmund Freud formulated the principles of psychoanalysis, emphasising the dramatic break of his ideas with what had gone before. Others locate the origin of psychotherapy at the moment Dubois (1905, 1906, 1909) formulated the principles of rational or moral therapy, or the time Pierre Janet (1901, 1907, 1924, 1925) started experimenting with hypnosis and suggestion around the turn of the twentieth century. Such histories correctly identify the historical moment that physicians appropriated and transformed culturally specific narrative practices, and articulated medical rationales for their approach to psychotherapy which were accompanied by claims of novelty and originality. These histories reflect attempts at professionalisation. Jones's (1953–1957) highly selective biography of Freud highlighted Freud's originality and downplayed his predecessors (Maddox, 2013). Such histories illustrate the functions and uses of disciplinary history (Graham, Lepenies, & Weingart, 1983) that accompany attempts to create a new profession by identifying pioneers, insiders, outsiders and potential heretics.

Historians, bound by different professional imperatives, have located the origins of psychotherapy much earlier. Ellenberger's (1970) magisterial study of the history of psychoanalysis analysed various developments in Continental thought evincing ideas that Freud would later incorporate in his formulations of the nature of the unconscious. Foucault (1978) argues that modern psychotherapy originated in the confession rituals of the Catholic church. He also highlighted the imperative to detect, identify and neutralise sexual impulses, which was already present in the writing of St. Augustine. Others have pointed to the various forms of pastoral care provided by representatives of religious groups for many centuries. The history of psychotherapy as a way of talking, often in a dyadic configuration characterised by an explicit asymmetry in roles, has a long history, primarily associated with religious forms of care for believers. Despite psychotherapists' objections that their techniques are scientifically neutral, pastoral care and psychotherapy are each other's repressed alter egos or doubles, as Borch-Jacobsen (1992) would describe it. In many ways, psychotherapy is a secularised form of pastoral care which incorporates many of its styles and promises similar redemptive qualities (Miller, this issue).

The history of various forms of psychotherapy in the North Atlantic has received ample attention, even though its historiography still contains significant gaps (Marks, 2017). Following Chakrabarthy (2000), it is necessary to provincialise the Northern Atlantic – Europe and North America – to identify the unusual and at times highly specific cultural repertoires that have subsumed modern forms of psychotherapy as it travelled across the globe. During the last three decades, physicians and professionals active in global mental health, eager to reduce the treatment gap for various forms of mental disorder in the developing world, have exported North Atlantic psychotherapeutic techniques wholesale to the rest of the world. Much of this export has paid little attention to how psychotherapy can best be implemented in various local contexts. Others have engaged in extensive dialogue with local practitioners, developing psychotherapeutic approaches that reflect local understandings of selfhood, distress and suffering. The dissemination of psychotherapy beyond the North Atlantic, before and after the launching of global mental health initiatives, has thus far received scant attention from historians. To study the spread of psychotherapy in the non-Western world, they need to form alliances with sociologists and anthropologists (Farmer, Kim, Kleinman, & Basilico, 2013). Because of its purported potency (Layard & Clark, 2015), the world-wide transfer and appropriation of psychotherapy deserves much more attention from scholars analysing the history, present state and possible futures of psychotherapy. We need to shift our attention from Europe and North America to what is often derisively called the 'Rest of the World.'

Psychotherapy in North America

Not only does psychotherapy appear to be more popular in North America than elsewhere, but historians have also studied its history and antecedent practices to a much greater extent there than anywhere else. A start to provincialising the North Atlantic can be made by analysing European and North American forms of psychotherapy as unusual and specific expressions of a broader genre, and by relating these to specific cultural influences that do not exist elsewhere. Cognitive-Behavioural Therapy, Albert Ellis' Rational-Emotive Therapy, and Aaron Beck's Cognitive Therapy had significant precursors in various advocates of positive thinking (Meyer, 1988) and various Protestant denominations (Caplan, 1998; Hale, 1971). These have inspired the turn of American psychoanalysis towards ego psychology (Hale, 1995) and away from the exploration of the unconscious and infantile sexuality, which both have been derided so eloquently by Jacques Lacan (1953/1996).

Aaron Beck's Rational Therapy, together with other forms of cognitive therapies, shows the possible effects of the transplantation of psychoanalysis from Europe to North America. Beck's self-styled 'splendid isolation,' as mentioned by Rachael Rosner (this issue), is an appealing figure of speech that places psychoanalysis, other developments within the world of American psychotherapy, and significant antecedents in the background while presenting cognitive psychotherapy as the sole invention of an individual mind. The excitement of Beck's collaborators embarking on an entirely new and innovative venture constitutes an interesting form of laboratory folklore, which might be partly based on a form of re-enactment or repetition of earlier, deeply ingrained American repertoires of addressing the ills that beset the mind. As Rosner emphasises, manualising psychotherapy and subjecting it to rigorous scientific analysis are specific to the North American context. Nevertheless, as she argues, the notion that psychotherapy essentially constitutes an art persists, and exists in an uneasy tension with scientific and rational approaches. Psychotherapy can never be fully manualised.

Psychotherapy in Europe's borderlands

Scotland, an area within the North Atlantic but far removed from its metropolitan academic and administrative centres such as Paris, Berlin, Vienna, London, New York and Boston, provides an interesting starting point for the provincialisation of dominant forms of psychotherapy. As Miller (this issue) argues, Scottish practitioners appropriated psychotherapy and incorporated it into specifically Scottish forms of Protestant thought and practice. Miller argues that both ministers and practitioners of psychotherapy considered it part of a constructive critique of Scottish Protestantism which could potentially remove undesirable elements such as supernaturalism and moralism. Unlike some early followers of psychoanalysis, who appreciated its ability to debunk religious superstition (see, for example, Heller and Rudnick (1991)), Scottish practitioners saw the capacity of psychotherapy to improve religious practice. They did not see religion as a form of wish-fulfilment or regression as other psychoanalysts did; they hoped to eliminate infantile impulses within it to arrive at a purer and more authentic religious practice.

Despite this belief that psychotherapy would strengthen religion, it probably contributed to its decline in association with wider processes of secularisation. Nonetheless, as Miller emphasises, the specifically Christian structure of life narratives (emphasising conversion experiences, devotion, and temptation) remained intertwined with Scottish psychotherapy. It is therefore not meaningful to analyse which elements in Scottish psychotherapy derive from various psychotherapeutic approaches and which from Scottish Protestantism. It is much more fruitful to rather investigate how it resulted from the deliberate intermingling of the two, before and after secularisation. Christianity may have declined but the ways in which it structured life narratives persist. It is possible to argue that typical Christian structures of life narratives have been appropriated by psychotherapists who presented them in the naturalistic language of psychology. Subsequently, Christian practitioners connected these life narratives with their erstwhile religious origins, after which they became separated again. Seen this way, religion and psychotherapy appear as intimately related rather antithetical.

Eastern Europe provides a very different but equally fruitful vantage point to analyse the inflections of psychotherapy in the European borderlands. Eastern Europe was located at a relatively short distance from Europe's metropolitan centres, yet the transformation of psychotherapeutic discourse and practice to the Communist sphere are distinct. Various authors (such as Etkind, 1997; Miller, 1998; Zajicek, 2014) have analysed the course of psychoanalysis and psychotherapy in the Soviet Union. Others have investigated the history of both in the German Democratic Republic (Eghigian, 2015; Leuenberger, 2001) and in eastern Europe in general (see the various contributors to Savelli and Marks (2015)). The initial enthusiasm in eastern Europe for psychoanalysis faded after Stalin dismissed it as a bourgeois fad upon his assumption of power. Sarah Marks (this issue) argues that, contrary to expectation, group therapy and labour therapy were not overly popular in eastern Europe. Instead, suggestion and persuasion continued to dominate psychotherapeutic approaches. Similarly, the influence of Paul Dubois was endured longer in eastern Europe than in western Europe and North America. After the development of various forms of cognitive psychotherapy, rational and cognitive approaches were popular in both the 'East' and the 'West', despite the vast political and ideological differences between the two.

Psychotherapy around the globe

Around the turn of the twentieth century, psychotherapists were influenced by several Asian sources. Taylor (1999), who has analysed the various religious and spiritualist influences on American psychotherapy, pays special attention to Theosophy (itself an interesting hybrid of Eastern and Western thought) and the influence of Swami Vivekananda and others, including Paramahansa Yogananda and Maharishi Mahesh Yogi, who visited the United States during the late nineteenth and early twentieth century. The visit of Japanese Buddhist thinker D.T. Suzuki to the United States in 1957 is a later demonstration of the desire of Western psychoanalysts and psychotherapists to enrich their practice by learning from Eastern spiritual leaders (Fromm, Suzuki, & De Martino, 1960). The influence of Eastern thinkers on Western thought was profound, even if Western thinkers did not fully understand their ideas. The influence of these spiritual leaders highlights the importance of spirituality in the North Atlantic region after the decline of institutionalised religion. At the same time, as Christopher Harding (this issue) emphasises, Asian spiritual leaders have appropriated psychological terminology. Recently, psychological and spiritual discursive repertoires appear to mix and mingle freely, although sometimes uneasily, in both the East and the West, inspiring a psychologised spirituality or spiritual styles of psychotherapy. Mindfulness-based psychotherapies, which have become very popular recently, illustrates the blending of spirituality and psychology well.

Harding presents a fascinating account of Japanese psychiatrist Kosawa Heisaku and his attempts to integrate Freud's psychoanalysis with the teachings of Shin Buddhism. Harding notes the spatial separation of psychoanalytic sessions, conducted on the proverbial couch, and Buddhist conversations, which were held in a different room afterwards, presumably with Kosawa and his patients sitting on normal chairs. This intriguing arrangement might indicate that Kosawa thought psychoanalysis and Shin Buddhism could only be integrated to a certain extent, or that both could complement each other while remaining faithful to their respective principles. Kosawa's therapeutic set-up constitutes a fascinating hybrid approach. His attempts resemble those of many others, both Western religious individuals and Asian thinkers seeking to integrate psychoanalysis in the various religions common in their regions. In India, for example, Jagadish Chandra Bose and several other intellectuals attempted to relate psychoanalytic thought to various Hindu narratives (Hartnack, 2011; Nandy, 1995a, 1995b). Carl Gustav Jung's views on the collective unconscious provided strong encouragement to include specific Indian archetypes and narratives in psychoanalytic theorising. Kosawa's and Bose's hybrid forms of psychoanalysis illustrate the inherent malleability and flexibility of psychoanalytic ideas.

The malleability of psychoanalysis already became apparent during its first decades, when several of Freud disciples developed creative versions of psychoanalytic psychotherapy which often clashed with more orthodox versions.

Psychoanalysts employed strategies of self-marginalisation to highlight its exclusive and controversial nature (Bos, Park, & Pietikainen, 2005) as well as internal control mechanisms to identify and exclude heretics. When psychoanalysis acquired the appearance of a profession, several prominent psychoanalysts went to great lengths to reduce variability by standardising training and practice, and by excluding those individuals who, in their opinion, failed to follow their visions. Within Freud's circle, there were a number of bitter splits with practitioners who, for a range of reasons, failed to follow the master's teachings. Performing and celebrating authenticity required continuous recrimination, denigration, marginalisation and exclusion. By excluding 'heretics' and exerting increasing control over psychoanalytic societies, training and psychoanalytic practice, psychoanalysis became increasingly rigid and lost its original creative bent. As a consequence, originality could only found outside the gates. From the few accounts that detail Freud's psychoanalytic sessions (Kardiner, 1977; Wortis, 1954), it appears that the master himself repeatedly failed to follow psychoanalytic protocol.

Beyond psychotherapy: psychoanalytic cosmologies

When the psychoanalytic imagination moves beyond the intricacies of conducting psychotherapy and articulated broader cosmological views, including creative alterations of religious and mythological narratives as well as shared cultural beliefs, creative appropriations appear infinite. Mariano Ben Plotkin (Plotkin, 2002, 2003) has provided excellent histories of psychoanalysis in Argentina. Cristiana Facchinetti (this issue) extends this analysis to Brazil and focuses in particular on the way a small group of modernist intellectuals applied psychoanalytic thought to forge a new, nationalist narrative in the 1920s (see also Plotkin (2008) and several essays in Damousi and Plotkin (2008)). Members of the Brazilian *avant-garde* incorporated Brazil's 'primitive' and pre-European past in a national narrative in which miscegenation between European settlers and South America's original inhabitants was seen as the basis for national strength and pride, rather than a source of embarrassment or degeneration. They emphasised Brazil's unique ability to produce a synthesis of both. Instead of trying to catch up with Europe, which increasingly displayed symptoms of degeneration, the intellectuals urged Brazilians to celebrate their unique origins as a nation to guide their future. Alienation could be overcome by acknowledging the previously repressed elements of Brazil's national identity, thereby redeeming its origins, which had been repressed.

Several recent studies have highlighted the development of psychiatry, psychology and psychotherapy across the globe. Linstrum (2016) has analysed how psychological experimentation and theorising in the United Kingdom relied on practices and experiences in the British Empire. In an innovative collection of essays, Anderson, Jenson, and Keller (2011) provide an overview of the many entanglements of colonialism and psychoanalysis, often inspired by a preoccupation with the primitive and Freud's *Totem and Taboo*. The psychoanalyst Géza Róheim, for example, travelled to Central Australia to study Aborigines to shed light on the first stages of human development (Anderson, 2014; Damousi, 2011). With the exception of Japan, Asia is mostly absent in this special issue, despite the presence of several fascinating appropriations of psychotherapy in recent years. Huang (2014), for example, has recently analysed China's current psycho-boom, while Hoesterey (2015) has investigated the appropriation of American pop psychology by popular Muslim cleric Aa Gym (Kyai Haji Abdullah Gymnastiar).

Religion

Several articles in this special issue discuss the often uncanny ties between religion and psychoanalysis or psychotherapy. Maslow (1956, p. 10) once stated, with a not uncommon hubris:'The world will either be saved by the psychologists or it won't be saved at all.'Only recently, another psychologist, Wright (2017), has argued that mindfulness can save America. Psychotherapists often claim that they can improve well-being, bring about happiness, and realise modern forms of transcendence, which is to say that they can provide secularised redemption. The trope of the psychiatrist, psychologist, or psychotherapist occupying the niche vacated by priests, ministers, rabbis (and imams?) has been commonplace (Rieff, 1966; Riesman, 1950). These narratives might be appealing because of their bold assertions and broad historical reach, but they nevertheless fail to detail how psychology, psychiatry and psychotherapy replaced the multitude of American religious denominations. Following the suggestion by Miller (this issue), it is better to analyse how various forms of psychotherapy have appropriated religious narrative templates and presented them in naturalised forms.

O'Donnell (1985) has amply documented that many early American psychologists had aspired to enter the ministry before turning to psychology. Most pastoral counsellors, who probably constitute the largest number of individuals practicing psychotherapy, are obviously convinced that psychotherapy and religion were compatible. Harding (this issue) notes the extensive 'religion-psy' dialogue that took place in during the 1950s in the United States and elsewhere. The dialogue between Carl Rogers and Paul Tillich mentioned by him reveals the many similarities between religion and psychotherapy. Some time ago, I investigated the eager reception of psychology and psychotherapy among Catholics during the 1950s and 1960s in the Netherlands (Pols, 1988). Many more studies of this kind could be adduced. Pastor Oskar Pfister and Freud corresponded in a most amiable matter about psychoanalysis; the former's religious commitments were not an obstacle (Malony & North, 1979). In many respects, religion and psychotherapy have been deeply enmeshed. Jung's father, for example, was a pastor of the Swiss Reformed Church, which has undoubtedly influenced Jung's proclivity to combine spirituality, religion and psychoanalysis.

Conclusion

Defined as a form of verbal human interaction with unusual redemptive properties, psychotherapy has a long history and an infinite number of appearances in different social, national and cultural contexts. Because of this, historical, trans-cultural and trans-national research on the many appearances of psychotherapy is unusually interesting. When they are transferred to new cultural spheres, psychotherapeutic practices evolve by incorporating novel cultural repertoires and narrative templates, and by discarding elements that are incompatible with shared cultural understandings. In the genealogy of psychotherapy, various interactions between thinkers from the East and West took place, which indicates that psychotherapy is not an exclusively Western invention. In the North Atlantic, a large number of variations and adaptions have been formulated and developed. Because of the dissemination of psychotherapeutic techniques across the globe, additional variations and innovations have been proposed. To chart the trans-cultural dissemination of psychotherapy, it is necessary to view its many European and North American forms as special cases. Viewing them as constitutive practices will inevitably portray novel and creative developments in the rest of the world as derivative. In our current era of global mental health (Collins et al., 2011; Patel, 2003; Patel, Minas, Cohen, & Prince, 2013), it can be expected that further variations will be developed.

Scholars have evaluated the social effect of psychotherapy's widespread acceptance differently. Hillman and Ventura (1993) have argued that the world continues to get worse despite the presence of 100 years of psychotherapy – a practice, they assert, that encourages individuals to focus on their inner woes and neglect social and political issues. These arguments are, of course, not entirely new and have been presented by others (Bellah, Madsen, Sullivan, Swidler, & Tipton, 1985; Furedi, 2004; Lasch, 1979; Putnam, 2001). Apart from being seen as a way of encouraging mildly alienated individuals to retreat to the comfortable world of middle class subjectivity, psychotherapy has been viewed as an essential tool for the counter-culture movement of the 1960s, the feminist movement, and the civil rights movement (Herman, 1995; Markowitz & Rosner, 1996). Psychotherapy appears to be capable of both encouraging and dampening social and political commitments. Its increasing penetration of the global world can stimulate a variety of social political developments, which should have the keen attention of psychotherapists, historians and social commentators.

Despite the apparent continued acclaim of psychotherapy, it will be important to focus on countervailing forces that could potentially undermine it, reduce its appeal, or replace it. After the introduction of anti-depressant medications in the 1990s, physicians and patients enthusiastically embraced this chemical cure for mental ills (Kramer, 1993). Following the mapping of the human genome and the decade of the brain, research in psychiatry has decidedly moved away from investigating the effects of psychotherapy in favour of exploring the genetic and other biological determinants of mental disorders. These new trends have shaped the way individuals view mental disorder (Dumit, 2004; Jenkin, 2010). The popular appeal of these psychopharmacological and neurological narratives is unusually powerful, which may enable them to replace the cognitive and affective narratives related to psychotherapy. It is possible that the present moment, as the popularity of psychotherapy threatens to be eclipsed by novel traditions from psychiatry and medicine, presents a significant opportunity to chart the courses of psychotherapy across the world over the last several centuries.

Apart from analysing the changing nature of psychotherapy when it enters new cultural domains, I would like to encourage psychotherapists to investigate the role of their profession within broader social, political and economic contexts as well. Some time ago, and with some overstatement, Albee (1990) highlighted the 'futility of psychotherapy' in modern societies that continuously impart neuroses in their citizens. He revived the ideals of the mental hygiene and mental health movements, which emphasised prevention, structural interventions, and the promotion of mental health over individualised treatment (Pols, 2007, 2010). Mental hygienists articulated a public health perspective on mental health. Physicians have been debating these issues under the banner of public health, international health, global health and planetary health (Boyden, 1995; McMichael, 2017) for over a century; psychiatrists, psychologists and other mental health professionals have done so to a more limited extent. For example, at the influential Alma Ata conference, organised in 1978 by the World Health Organisation, physicians advocated access to health care as a human right and discussed issues of social justice (Litsios, 2002). According to the Ottawa charter for Health Promotion, formulated as a follow-up to this conference, the fundamental conditions for health are peace, shelter, education, food, income, a stable eco-system, sustainable resources, social justice and equity (World Health Organization, 1986). It is not unreasonable to assume that the conditions outlined in the Ottawa charter are also fundamental to mental health.

There has been ample research on mental health that could potentially inspire public mental health perspectives. The path-breaking study of Hollingshead and Redlich (1958) established a strong correlation between poverty and severe and persistent forms of mental illness. It also presented a paradox central to mental health care: most mental health expenditure (both public and private) supports the less severe ills of individuals in the highest socio-economic classes while less funding is available for the treatment of the severe and persistent forms of mental illness in the poor. With inequality growing at an unprecedented rate in North America and Asia, this situation is worsening (Alvaredo, Chancel, Piketty, Saez, & Zucman, 2017). Unfortunately, psychologists, psychiatrists and psychotherapists have, often implicitly, blamed the poor by developing theories on the personal causes of their poverty (Raz, 2016). Apart from advocates of ecopsy-chology (Kahn & Hasbach, 2012; Nemeth, Hamilton, & Kuriansky, 2015; Roszak, Gomes, & Kanner, 1995), psychotherapists have addressed the consequences of climate change and environmental degradation on mental health only to a limited extent. In addition to investigating the ramifications of the transmission of psychotherapy between cultures, as the authors in this special issue have done in a fascinating way, I would encourage psychotherapists to continue analysing the place of psychotherapy in broader social and political contexts.

Disclosure statement

No potential conflict of interest was reported by the author.

References

Albee, G. W. (1990). The futility of psychotherapy. *Journal of Mind and Behavior, 11*(3/4), 369–384.

Alvaredo, F., Chancel, L., Piketty, T., Saez, E., & Zucman, G. (2017). *World inequality report 2018*. Paris: World Inequality Lab.

Anderson, W. (2014). Hermannsburg, 1929: Turning aboriginal "primitives" into modern psychological subjects. *Journal of the History of the Behavioral Sciences, 50*(2), 127–147.

Anderson, W., Jenson, D., & Keller, R. (2011). *Unconscious dominions: Psychoanalysis, colonial trauma, and global sovereignties*. Durham, NC: Duke University Press.

Bellah, R. N., Madsen, R., Sullivan, W. M., Swidler, A., & Tipton, S. M. (1985). *Habits of the heart: Individualism and commitment in American life*. New York, NY: Harper & Row.

Borch-Jacobsen, M. (1992). *The emotional tie: Psychoanalysis, mimesis, and affect*. Stanford, CA: Stanford University Press.

Bos, J., Park, D. W., & Pietikainen, P. (2005). Strategic self-marginalization: The case of psychoanalysis. *Journal of the History of Behavioral Sciences, 41*(3), 207–224.

Boyden, S. (1995). *The biology of civilisation: Understanding human culture as a force in nature*. Sydney: University of New South Wales Press.

Caplan, E. (1998). *Mind games: American culture and the birth of psychotherapy*. Berkeley: University of California Press.

Chakrabarthy, D. (2000). *Provincializing Europe*. Princeton, NJ: Princeton University Press.

Collins, P. Y., Patel, V., Joestl, S. S., March, D., Insel, T. R., & Daar, A. S. (2011). Grand challenges in global mental health. *Nature, 475*, 27–30.

Damousi, J. (2011). Géza Róheim and the Australian Aborigine psychoanalytic anthropology during the interwar years. In W. Anderson, D. Jenson, & R. C. Keller (Eds.),

Unconscious dominions: Psychoanalysis, colonial trauma, and global sovereignties (pp. 75–96). Durnham, NC: Duke University Press.

Damousi, J., & Plotkin, M. (2008). *The transnational unconscious: Essays in the history of psychoanalysis and transnationalism*. New York, NY: Palgrave MacMillan.

Dubois, P. (1905). *The psychic treatment of nervous disorders: The psychoneuroses and their moral treatment* (S. E. Jelliffe & W. A. White, Trans.). New York, NY: Funk & Wagnalls.

Dubois, P. (1906). *The influence of the mind on he body* (L. B. Gallatin, Trans.). New York, NY: Funk & Wagnalls.

Dubois, P. (1909). *Self-control and how to secure it* (H. H. Boyd, Trans.). New York, NY: Funk & Wagnalls.

Dumit, J. (2004). *Picturing personhood: Brain scans and biomedical identity*. Princeton, NJ: Princeton University Press.

Eghigian, G. (2015). *The corrigible and the incorrigible: Science, medicine, and the convict in twentieth-century Germany*. Ann Arbor, MI: University of Michigan Press.

Ellenberger, H. F. (1970). *The discovery of the unconscious: The history and evolution of dynamic psychiatry*. New York, NY: Basic.

Etkind, A. M. (1997). *Eros of the impossible: The history of psychoanalysis in Russia* (N. a. M. Rubens, Trans.). Boulder, CO: Westview Press.

Farmer, P., Kim, J. Y., Kleinman, A., & Basilico, M. (Eds.). (2013). *Reimagining global heatlh: An introduction*. Berkeley, CA: California University Press.

Foucault, M. (1978). *The history of sexuality: An Introduction* (R. Hurley, Trans. Vol. 1). New York, NY: Pantheon.

Fromm, E., Suzuki, D. T., & De Martino, R. (1960). *Zen Buddhism and psychoanalysis*. New York, NY: Harper & Row.

Furedi, F. (2004). *Therapy culture: Cultivating vulnerability in an uncertain age*. London: Routledge.

Graham, L., Lepenies, W., & Weingart, P. (1983). *Functions and uses of disciplinary history*. Dordrecht: Reidel.

Hale, N. G. (1971). *The beginnings of psychoanalysis in the United States, 1876–1917*, Vol. 1. New York, NY: Oxford University Press.

Hale, N. G. (1995). *The rise and crisis of psychoanalysis in the United States, 1917–1985*, Vol. 2. New York, NY: Oxford Univ Press.

Hartnack, C. (2011). Colonial dominions and the psychoanalytic couch: Synergies of Freudian theory with Bengali Hindu thought and practices in British India. In W. H. Anderson, D. Jenson, & R. Keller (Eds.), *Unconscious dominions: Psychoanalysis, colonial trauma, and global sovereignties* (pp. 141–165). Durham, NC: Duke University Press.

Heller, A. & Rudnick, L. (Eds.). (1991). *1915, the cultural moment: The new politics, the new woman, the new psychology, the new art, and the new theatre in America*. New Brunswick, NJ: Rutgers University Press.

Herman, E. (1995). *The romance of American psychology: Political culture in the age of experts*. Berkeley: University of California Press.

Hillman, J., & Ventura, M. (1993). *We've had a hundred years of psychotherapy: And the world's getting worse*. New York, NY: HarperOne.

Hoesterey, J. B. (2015). *Rebranding Islam: Piety, prosperity, and a self-help guru*. Stanford, CA: Stanford University Press.

Hollingshead, A. B., & Redlich, F. C. (1958). *Social class and mental illness: A community study*. New York, NY: Wiley.

Huang, H.-Y. (2014). The emergence of the psycho-boom in contemporary China. In H. Chiang (Ed.), *Psychiatry and Chinese history* (pp. 183–204). London: Pickering & Chatto.

Janet, P. (1901). *The mental states of hystericals: A study of mental stigmata and mental accidents* (C. R. Corson, Trans.). New York, NY: Putnam.

Janet, P. (1907). *The major symptoms of hysteria*. New York, NY: MacMillan.

Janet, P. (1924). *Principles of psychotherapy* (H. M. a. E. R. Guthrie, Trans.). New York, NY: MacMillan.

Janet, P. (1925). *Psychological healing: A historical and clinical study* (E. P. C. Paul, Trans.). New York, NY: MacMillan.

Jenkin, J. H. (Ed.). (2010). *Pharmaceutical self: The global shaping of experience in an age of psychopharmacology*. Santa Fe, NM: SAR Press.

Jones, E. (1953–1957). *The life and work of Sigmund Freud*. New York, NY: Basic Books.

Kahn, P. H., Jr & Hasbach, P. H. (Eds.). (2012). *Ecopsychology: Science, totems, and the technological species*. Cambridge, MA: MIT Press.

Kardiner, A. (1977). *My analysis with Freud: Reminiscences*. New York, NY: Norton.

Kramer, P. D. (1993). *Listening to prozac: A psychiatrist explores antidepressant drugs and the remaking of the self*. New York, NY: Penguin.

Lacan, J. (1953/1996). The function and field of speech and language in psychoanalysis (B. Fink, Trans.). In *Écrits: A selection* (pp. 197–268). New York, NY: Norton.

Lasch, C. (1979). *The culture of narcissim: American life in an age of diminishing expectations*. New York, NY: Norton.

Latour, B. (1990). Drawing things together. In M. Lynch & S. Woolgar (Eds.), *Representation in scientific practice* (pp. 19–68). Cambridge: MIT Press.

Layard, R., & Clark, D. M. (2015). *Thrive: The power of evidence-based psychological therapies*. London: Penguin.

Leuenberger, C. (2001). Socialist psychotherapy and its dissidents. *Journal of the History of the Behavioural Sciences, 37*, 267–373.

Linstrum, E. (2016). *Ruling minds: Psychology in the British empire*. Cambridge: Harvard University Press.

Litsios, S. (2002). The long and difficult road to Alma-Ata: A personal reflection. *International Journal of Health Services, 32*, 709–732.

Maddox, B. (2013). *Freud's wizard: Ernest Jones and the transformation of psychoanalysis*. New York, NY: Da Capo.

Malony, N., & North, G. (1979). The future of an illusion – the illusion of the future an historic dialogue on the value of religion between Oskar Pfister and Sigmund Freud. *Journal of the History of the Behavioral Sciences, 15*(2), 177–186.

Markowitz, G., & Rosner, D. (1996). *Children, race, and power: Kenneth and Mamie Clark's Northside Center*. Charlottesville, VA: University Press of Virginia.

Marks, S. (2017). Psychotherapy in historical perspective. *History of the Human Sciences, 30*(2), 3–16.

Maslow, A. H. (1956). Toward a humanistic psychology. *ETC: A Review of General Semantics, 14*(1), 10–22.

McMichael, A. (2017). *Climate change and the health of nations: Famines, fevers, and the fate of populations*. Oxford: Oxford University Press.

Meyer, D. B. (1988). *The positive thinkers: Popular religious psychology from Mary Baker Eddy to Norman Vincent Peale and Ronald Reagan*. Middletown, CT: Wesleyan University Press.

Miller, M. A. (1998). *Freud and the Bolsheviks: Psychoanalysis in imperial Russia and the Soviet Union*. New Haven, CT: Yale University Press.

Nandy, A. (1995a). *Alternative sciences: Creativity and authenticity in two Indian scientists*. Oxford: Oxford University Press.

Nandy, A. (1995b). *The savage Freud and other essays on possible and retrievable selves*. Princeton, NJ: Princeton University Press.

Nemeth, D. G., Hamilton, R. B., & Kuriansky, J. (2015). *Ecopsychology: Advances from the intersection of psychology and environmental protection*. Santa Barbara, CA: Praeger.

O'Donnell, J. M. (1985). *The origins of behaviorism: American psychology, 1870–1920*. New York, NY: New York University Press.

Patel, V. (2003). *Where there is no psychiatrist: A mental health care manual*. London: Gaskell.

Patel, V., Minas, H., Cohen, A., & Prince, H. J. (2013). *Global mental health: Principles and practice*. New York, NY: Oxford University Press.

Plotkin, M. B. (2002). *Freud in the pampas: The emergence and development of a psychoanalytic culture in Argentina*. Stanford, CA: Stanford University Press.

Plotkin, M. B. (2003). *Argentina on the couch: Psychiatry, state, and society, 1880 to the present*. Albuquerque, NM: University of New Mexico Press.

Plotkin, M. B. (2008). Psychoanalysis, transnationalism and national habitus: A comparative approach to the reception of psychoanalysis in Argentina and Brazil (1910s–1940s). In J. Damousi & M. Plotkin (Eds.), *The transnational Unconscious: Essays in the history of psychoanalysis and transnationalism* (pp. 145–176). New York, NY: Palgrave MacMillan.

Pols, H. (1988). Genezen van de moraal: Over Katholieken en de geestelijke gezondheidszorg in Nederland, 1930–1950. *Kennis & Methode, 12*(1), 4–21.

Pols, H. (2007). Frankwood E. Williams on finding a way in mental hygiene. *American Journal of Public Health, 96*(4), 616–619.

Pols, H. (2010).'Beyond the clinical frontiers': The mental hygiene movement in the United States. In V. Roelcke, P. J. Weindling, & L. Westwood (Eds.), *International relations in psychiatry: Britain, Germany, and the United States to world war II* (pp. 111–133). Rochester, NY: Rochester University Press.

Putnam, R. D. (2001). *Bowling alone: The collapse and revival of American community*. New York, NY: Simon & Schuster.

Raz, M. (2016). *What's wrong with the poor?: Psychiatry, race, and the war on poverty*. Durham: University of North Carolina Press.

Rieff, P. (1966). *The triumph of the therapeutic: Uses of faith after Freud*. New York, NY: Harper.

Riesman, D. (1950). *The lonely crowd: A study of the changing American character*. New Haven, CT: Yale University Press.

Roszak, T., Gomes, M. E., & Kanner, A. D. (Eds.). (1995). *Ecopsychology: Restoring the earth, healing the mind*. San Francisco, CA: Sierra Club Books.

Savelli, M., & Marks, S. (2015). *Psychiatry in communist Europe*. Basingstoke Hampshire: Palgrave MacMillan.

Taylor, E. (1999). *Shadow culture: Psychology and spirituality in America*. Washington, DC: Counterpoint.

World Health Organization (1986). *Ottawa charter for health promotion*. Geneva: Author.

Wortis, J. (1954). *Fragments of an analysis with Freud*. New York, NY: Simon and Schuster.

Wright, R. (2017, 10 August). How mindfullness can save America *WIRED*. Retrieved December 9, 2017 from https://www.wired.com/story/how-mindful-meditation-can-save-us-from-the-tribal-abyss/

Zajicek, B. (2014). Soviet Madness: nervousness, mild schizophrenia, and the professional jurisdiction of psychiatry in the USSR, 1918–1936. *Ab Imperio, 4*, 167–194.

Transcultural histories of psychotherapy

Keir Martin [iD]

ABSTRACT
Both proponents of and critics tend to assume psychotherapy's origin and status as a 'Western' practice. The history of the emergence of psychoanalysis and psychotherapy are far more complex than this picture allows for. Today as we enter a more multipolar era of world history, the easy identification of psychotherapy with 'the West' will become increasingly difficult to sustain, as Bangalore and Shanghai are likely to rival Hampstead and Manhattan as centres of influence for the development of therapeutic practice and theory in the coming decades. Adapting to this new world will necessitate a different conception of the role of 'culture' than we have been used to in recent discussions in psychotherapy. Rather than simply seeing 'culture' as a factor that needs to be added to discussions to counteract the alleged ethnocentrism of 'Western' psychotherapy, we will need to begin to pay more careful attention to the work that is done by appeals to the 'culture concept' in different contexts. In particular 'culture' can be constructed as an object of evaluation that makes it part of the 'check-list' of skills that characterise the reconception of psychotherapy in an era of neoliberal instrumental manualised therapy training and practice.

Historias Transculturales En Psicoterapia

Los proponents y los críticos de la universalidad de las teorías psicoterapéuticas, tienden a asumir sus orígenes y su 'status' como una práctica occidental. La historia del surgimiento del psicoanálisis y de la psicoterapia es mucho más compleja de lo que esta postura permite; por otra parte, su gran aceptación es en muy buena parte el resultado de la unipolaridad en el orden politico-económico de principios del siglo XX, en el cual estas disciplinas comenzaron a desarrollarse. En el presente, el balance global de la influencia politico-económica ha cambiado y entramos en una era de la historia mundial más unipolar, en la cual una identificación de la psicoterapia con "el Oeste" llegaría a ser muy difícil de sostener desde un punto de vista analítico. Incluso,si las historias de los orígenes de la psicoterapia no se escriben de nuevo, Bangalore y Shanghai pueden llegar a rivalizar con Hampstead y Manhattan como centros de influencia en el desarrollo de la teoría y práctica de la psicoterapia en las décadas venideras. Para adaptarnos a este nuevo mundo, será necesaria una concepción del role de la cultura diferente a la que ha sido utilizada en discusiones recientes acerca de la psicoterapia. En lugar de ver "la cultura" como un factor que necesita añdirse a las discusiones para contrarrestar un reconocido etnocentrismo en la psicoterapia occidental, necesitamos comenzar a prestar atención al trabajo realizado por la atracción que ofrece el concepto "cultura" en diferentes contextos. La cultura, particularmente, puede ser construida como un objeto de evaluación que la hace parte de una "lista a chequear" de habilidades que caracterizan la re-concepción de la psicoterapia, en una era neo-liberal en la cual, la formación y la práctica de la psicoterapia parecen marchar hacia su instrumentalización manualizada.

Storie transculturali della psicoterapia

Sia i fautori che i critici dell'universalità cross-culturale delle teorie psicoterapeutiche ne condividono l'origine e lo status di pratica "occidentale". Tuttavia, la storia della nascita della psicoanalisi e psicoterapia che ne deriva sono molto più complesse di quanto questa visione consenta: la sua diffusa accettazione è il risultato di un ordinamento economico-politico unipolarizzato sull'occidente, caratteristico del primo Novecento. Oggi l'equilibrio globale dato dalla politica e dall'economia si è spostato ed entriamo in un'era più "multipolare" della storia del mondo; anche la semplicistica identificazione della psicoterapia con "l'Occidente" sarà sempre più difficile da sostenere. Benché le storie delle origini della psicoterapia non vengano riscritte, Bangalore e Shanghai probabilmente saranno in competizione con Hampstead e Manhattan quali centri d'influenza per lo sviluppo della pratica terapeutica e della teoria psicoanalitica nei prossimi decenni. Adattarsi a questo nuovo mondo richiederà una diversa concezione del ruolo giocato dalla "cultura", rispetto a ciò a cui siamo abituati nelle dissertazioni sulla psicoterapia. Piuttosto che vedere semplicemente la "cultura" come un fattore aggiuntivo nelle discussioni per contrastare il presunto etnocentrismo della psicoterapia "occidentale", dovremo iniziare a prestare maggiore attenzione agli appelli al "concetto cultura" in diversi contesti. In particolare, la "cultura" può essere costruita come oggetto di valutazione che la rende parte della "lista di controllo" delle abilità che caratterizzano la ri-concezione della psicoterapia in un'epoca di formazione e pratica terapeutica strumentale neoliberista.

Histoires transculturelles de la psychothérapie

Les défenseurs tout comme les opposants de l'universalité transculturelle des théories psychothérapeutiques tendent à supposer leur origine et leur statut comme une pratique occidentale. L'histoire de l'émergence de la psychanalyse et de la psychothérapie est plus complexe qu'il n'y paraît et leur acceptation généralisée est aussi le résultat d'un ordre économique politique occidental unipolaire du début du 20ième siècle au sein duquel elles se sont développées. De nos jours l'équilibre des influences politiques et économiques se modifiant, nous entrons dans une ère davantage multipolaire de l'histoire du monde où l'identification facile de la psychothérapie avec l'Occident deviendra de plus en plus difficile à soutenir comme point de départ analytique. Même si l'histoire des origines de la psychothérapie ne sera pas réécrite, Bangalore et Shanghai sont en passe de rivaliser avec Hampstead et Manhattan en tant que centres d'influence du développement de la pratique et de la théorie psychothérapeutiques dans les décennies à venir. S'adapter à ce nouveau monde nécessitera une conception différente du rôle de « la culture » auquel nous avons été habitués lors des récentes discussions autour de la psychothérapie. Plutôt que de simplement voir «la culture » comme facteur devant être ajouté aux discussions afin de contrebalancer le caractère ethnocentrique de la psychothérapie occidentale, nous devrons commencer à faire plus attention au travail qui est fait en référence au « concept de culture » dans différents contextes. En particulier «la culture» qui peut être construite comme un objet d'évaluation venant l'ajouter à la liste des compétences caractérisant la re-conception de la psychothérapie dans une ère néolibérale où les pratiques et les formations en psychothérapie tendent à être instrumentalisées et manualisées.

Διαπολιτισμικές ιστορίες της ψυχοθεραπείας

ΠΕΡΙΛΗΨΗ

Τόσο οι υποστηρικτές, όσο και οι επικριτές της υπόθεσης ότι οι ψυχοθεραπευτικές θεωρίες είναι διαπολιτισμικά οικουμενικές έχουν την τάση να θεωρούν την προέλευση και τη θέση της ψυχοθεραπείας ως «δυτική» πρακτική. Η ιστορία της ανάδυσης της ψυχανάλυσης και της ψυχοθεραπείας είναι πολύ πιο πολύπλοκη και η ευρεία αποδοχή αυτής της άποψης είναι εξίσου κατά κύριο λόγο (βγάζει πιο πολύ νόημα)αποτέλεσμα της μονόπλευρης δυτικής πολιτικής οικονομικής τάξης που επικρατούσε στις αρχές του 20ου αιώνα, όταν εδραιώθηκε η ψυχοθεραπεία. Σήμερα, καθώς η παγκόσμια ισορροπία των πολιτικών και οικονομικών επιδράσεων μεταβάλλεται και εισερχόμαστε σε μια εποχή της παγκόσμιας ιστορίας που χαρακτηρίζεται από πολλαπλά κέντρα εξουσίας, οη εύκολη ταύτιση της ψυχοθεραπείας με «τη Δύση» θα γίνεται όλο και πιο δύσκολο να διατηρηθεί ως αναλυτικό σημείο εκκίνησης. Ακόμη και αν η ιστορία της προέλευσης της ψυχοθεραπείας δεν ξαναγραφεί, είναι πιθανό ότι στις επόμενες δεκαετίες η Bangalore και η Shanghai θα ανταγωνίζονται το Hampstead και το Manhattan ως κέντρα επιρροής στην ανάπτυξη της θεραπευτικής πρακτικής και θεραπείας. Η προσαρμογή σε αυτό τον νέο κόσμο θα απαιτήσει μια διαφορετική αντίληψη του ρόλου του πολιτισμού από αυτή που είχαμε συνηθίσει στις μέχρι πρόσφατα συζητήσεις για τη ψυχοθεραπεία. Αντί να αντιμετωπίζουμε «τον πολιτισμό» απλώς ως έναν παράγοντα που χρειάζεται να λαμβάνεται υπόψη ώστε να αντισταθμίζεται ο εθνοκεντρισμός της «δυτικής ψυχοθεραπείας», χρειάζεται να αρχίσουμε να δίνουμε περισσότερη προσοχή σε αυτό που επιτυγχάνεται μέσω της έκκλησης στην «έννοια του πολιτισμού» σε διαφορετικά πλαίσια. Πιο συγκεκριμένα, ο πολιτισμός μπορεί να κατασκευάζεται ως ένα αντικείμενο αξιολόγησης, που την καθιστά μέρος της λίστας ελέγχου των δεξιοτήτων που θεωρείται ότι πρέπει να διαθέτει ένας θεραπευτής στην αναδιατύπωση της ψυχοθεραπείας στην εποχή της νεοφιλελεύθερης συντελεστικής εκπαίδευσης και της πρακτικής της θεραπείας με βάση εγχειρίδια.

Introduction

Whether or not the perspectives given on the human condition by 'psychotherapy' in its various manifestations are universal truths or particular cultural perspectives, its historic origin as a 'Western' discipline is largely assumed by advocates and opponents alike. In the popular imagination, not only analysis but psychotherapy more generally is often considered to have emerged with Freud and his circle in late nineteenth century Vienna, despite the precedents for a 'talking cure' for mental and emotional distress, that predated Freud and his contemporaries, and despite Freud's own careful use of the term psychoanalysis to distinguish his developing technique from other already established psychotherapies. Rightly or wrongly, the story of psychotherapy is often told in terms of a Freudian origin followed by a succession of schisms on a variety of grounds.

In this paper, I explore the extent to which psychotherapy's history really unproblematically qualifies it as a 'Western' practice. I argue instead that the triumph of this narrative largely reflects the unipolar Western centre of global political and economic power at the time of contemporary psychotherapy's emergence in the early twentieth century, and that this assumption is likely to be increasingly destabilised by a move to a more multipolar world in the twenty-first century. The irony is that many involved in the teaching and regulation of psychotherapy are moving towards a model of 'cultural competence' that is implicitly or explicitly based on the idea of separate bounded cultures, and that the work of psychotherapy as a 'Western' discipline is to demonstrate its ability to incorporate those other 'cultures' at the point when these underlying assumptions might be increasingly in the process of being undermined by global economic and political changes. In the second half of the paper, I explore the ways in which contemporary psychotherapy training has moved towards a 'manualised' skills-based approach, in which this conception of 'culture' as an object belonging to particular groups can be operationalised as a key skill or competence to demonstrate mastery of on a check-list. Hence even if the assumptions underpinning these 'cultural competence' models are being subverted by global changes, they are likely to retain their power as they fit a zeitgeist in therapy training that favours the demonstration of skills and techniques over personal development and meeting.

Psychotherapy and the claim to universal truth

Schisms within psychotherapy and related critiques from outside of the dis-cipline have had a number of bases of which one of the most enduring has been the criticism that Freudian (and other 'Western') psychotherapies assume a universalised vision of what it is (or ideally should be) to be human based on late nineteenth century middle-class Vienna (Freud), 1950s America (Rogers) or whatever 'Western' context the particular therapeutic model in question had emerged from. Ever since Ernest Jones' debates with Malinowski in the 1920s, the critique of the alleged universality of the Oedipus complex has provided ammunition for sceptical anthropologists keen to point out its alleged assump-tion of a particular kind of patriarchal bourgeois nuclear family in the face of evidence from other cultures that this is precisely what cannot be assumed. Subsequent interventions in anthropology (e.g. Obeysekere, 1990; Spiro, 1982) have tended towards the conclusion that, as Moore (2007, p. 140) observes there is now, 'a loose consensus that a 'family romance' in some sense must be universal, but that it's content is cross-culturally variable'. This disagreement over the relative limits of universalist versus culturalist explanations can in many ways be seen as the basis for an ongoing debate between the two disciplines (Moore, 2007, p. 137).

Although this cross-cultural critique would be expected from anthropology, it has a long provenance in other fields as well, not least from those outside of Europe who received the new doctrine with a mixture of enthusiasm and scepticism in the early years of the twentieth century. Not only was psychoanal-ysis turned against its own allegedly underpinning Eurocentric assumptions by political and cultural radicals from its early days, such as the Brazilian intellectual movements described in this volume by *Facchinetti*, but also by founding figures of non-Western psychoanalytic traditions. *Harding* describes the case of Kosawa Heisaku, in Japan, to whose example could be added that of Girindrasekhar Bose in India. Both men are considered founders of their national psychoanalytic traditions and both carried out a debate with Freud regarding the universality or variability of the Oedipus complex in their respective national contexts. Bose (1949) for example stated that in India, boys ideally do not develop either a desire for the mother or a fear of castration by the father, but rather a desire to be the mother and bear the father's children.

This tradition of nuanced cultural critique by those sympathetic to Freud, but rejecting the universalist dogmatism that Freud laid down for his followers, continued through the twentieth century. Decades after Bose, his successor as the major figure in Indian psychoanalysis, Kakar (1978) for example, also decon-structed Oedipus on the slightly different grounds that, for Indian boys their major developmental problem is a growing realisation that they cannot effec-tively meet the sexual needs that their mothers unconsciously communicate to them causing them to feel swamped, rather than the familiar sexual rivalry with the father of Freudian myth. As Akhtar and Tummala-Narra (2008, p. 3) observe however, such histories remain largely unknown to Western analysts for whom both the universal truth of and Western origin of much analytic theory still seems to go largely unquestioned regardless of potentially differing interpretations. Bose, for example, developed his own psychoanalytic practice and theory, partly based upon Hindu religious philosophy *before* he entered into correspondence with Freud, meaning that Indian psychoanalysis could well be considered to have developed, 'independently of Freud's direct personal influence' (Akhtar & Tummala-Narra, 2008, p. 3,8; Meckel, 2009, p. 214). As is well known, Freud's obsessive desire to stamp psychoanalysis as his own creation has helped to create an origin myth in which rival movements tend to be seen as outgrowths or splits rather than theories or perspectives in their own right. When Bose sent Freud a statue of Lord Vishnu for his 75th birthday, Freud wrote back to Bose, the author of his own independent psychoanalytic tradition, with warm thanks for the gift, adding that, '[A]s long as I enjoy life it will recall to my mind the progress of Psychoanalysis [,] the proud conquests it has made in foreign countries', (quoted in Ramana, 1964). This story of the Western origin and then foreign conquest and spread of psychoanalysis has become so well established that it is now conventional to think of psychoanalysis and psychotherapy as 'Western' technologies of the self even among those who seek to question its cross-cultural applicability.

A new global psychotherapy

Even if is too late to rewrite that questionable history, is it the case that events are overtaking it on the ground in a manner that will make models implicitly based upon the 'impact' or 'applicability' of (assumed) 'Western' therapeutic concepts and practices in 'non-Western' contexts increasingly obsolete? Part of the 'West's' seeming ownership of psychotherapy may be down to the aggressive claiming of primacy revealed by Freud's response to Bose's. This begs the question of why Freud was able to pull this particular stunt on Bose and not the other way around. In one of the classic texts of anthropological theory, Mauss (1925/1966), writing at around this time, in the 1920s, claims, in the context of a discussion of classical Indian civilisation, that an inability or failure to reciprocate the Gift wounds the recipient and reinscribes the hierarchical authority of the giver. In this case however, Freud's inability to fully reciprocate Bose's gift, that embodied the Hindu Indian cosmology underpinning Bose's very different psychoanalytic system, with anything other than a statement of his ownership of the whole project, was intended to reinscribe his authority at the donor's expense. That he was able to do so was not due to any greater scientific accuracy of his particular scheme but was instead a consequence of the unipolar world of that time.

This is the context in which the Brazilian cultural revolutionaries described by *Facchinetti* could accept that psychotherapy was a European technology and thereby set themselves the task of attempting to de-construct its inherent Westernness as part of a de-colonising cultural project. In other similar contexts psychoanalysis' perceived Europeanness would be appropriated in entirely the opposite direction. In neighbouring Argentina it was famously appropriated as an icon of that country's supposed greater degree of European modernity and a badge of Buenos Aires' status as the Paris of Latin America.

A century on and the world looks in many regards a very different place. Private psychotherapy has often been associated with a middle-class clientele that had the time and money to engage with it. In previous decades, the qualifying adjective 'Western' was often not needed before the term middle-class. The very emergence of such a group was frequently considered emblematic of a modernity that only the West had achieved. The middle-classes of the non-Western world tended (as with so many other phenomena) to be largely considered as marginal and to be evaluated by the extent to which they measured up to the already established Western template. The rapid shift away from this unipolar world to one with powerful political economic actors in previously marginal territories is potentially one of the biggest drivers of transcultural global change that the world has witnessed to date. According to the OECD the 'global middle class' will increase from 1.8bn in 2009, to 4.9bn by 2030 (Pezzini, 2012). Most of this growth is occurring in parts of the world that have previously not had a numerous middle-class. Asia's share of the global middle-class population is estimated to rise from 28 to 66% in this period, whilst Europe and North America's share is projected to fall by a similar degree (Pezzini, 2012). This development marks a historically unprecedented shift in the global economic and cultural balance of power, as the emerging middle-class of nations such as India and China become major new centres for the production of consumer demand and political influence. The Chinese middle class is predicted to take over from the US middle class as the main driver of global consumer demand within the next thirty years for example, (Kharas & Gertz, 2010). Although there is some debate over some of the claims as the growth of this sector of the world's population and the statistical methods used to substantiate these claims (e.g. Kochlar & Oates, 2015), few would deny that, the growth of the global middle-classes' is now a phenomenon of unavoidable scale and importance. For some, such as Peter Lindert, it is a political and cultural transformation that is far more historically impressive than the British Industrial Revolution that revolutionised the world two centuries previously (Lindert cited in Freehand, 2011).

Psychotherapy is emerging as an important technique by which members of the newly emerging middle class reshape their subjectivities, whilst at the same time psychotherapy as a cultural practice is itself being reshaped by its own role in this transformation. Psychotherapy's major role in reshaping Western society over the past century is well-documented (e.g. Madsen, 2014). There is little doubt that private psychotherapy is fast becoming one of the major locations in which the new global middle classes engage in such processes of personal recreation. Indeed, the unprecedented expansion of psychotherapy as an item of individual consumption and technique for self-improvement among the fast-growing middle classes is one of the clearest markers of the socio-economic developments discussed above. Across the so-called BRIC nations (Brazil, Russia, India and China), singled out as the leaders in this shift in economic and political influence similar tendencies can be observed. In Brazil, a 'significant increase' in individual uptake of psychotherapy is reported since around the turn of the millennium (Hutz & Gomes, 2013, p. 102), around the same time as poverty reduction programmes and economic growth are described as having led to a rapid jump in the size of the country's middle-class (Pezzini, 2012). In Russia, Matza (2012, p. 804) reports how psychotherapy has gone from being condemned as 'bourgeois "self-rummaging"' in the Soviet era to becoming a central part of how members of an emerging 'middle-class' strive to create themselves as, 'an autonomous neoliberal actor primed for competition' (Matza, 2012, p. 812). This has created a situation where, advertisements for counselling and psychotherapy now, 'dot the yellow pages' seeking to, 'cater to the quest for the extracurricular that has become a feature of global middle-class life', (Matza, 2012, pp. 804–805). In India the number of universities offering training in counselling and psychotherapy, predominantly designed to cater to this new middle-class clientele has expanded from 1 in 2001, to 25 in 2016 (Tony George, professor of psychology, Christ University Bangalore, personal communication). In China, Zhang (2016, p. 121) reports a rapid increase in the uptake of psychotherapy and other forms of 'psychological counselling among the Chinese middle-class urban residents'. This is in a context where, similarly to Russia, psychotherapy and counselling have gone from being denounced as a, 'useless or harmful bourgeois intervention' two decades ago to now being so mainstream that is estimated that 100,000 Chinese have certification as psychotherapy or counselling practitioners (Zhang, 2016) and psychotherapists are major television celebrities (Huang, 2015).

Most anthropological work on the introduction of psychotherapy in non-Western contexts has been in contexts such as the provision of therapy by aid organisations those considered to be at risk of trauma following natural disaster or political violence (e.g. Herman, 1992; Petty & Bracken, 1998; Young, 1995). The consequent prevailing analytic focus of such accounts has tended to be variants of the already established framing of psychotherapy as a fundamentally 'Western' theory and practice. These tend to be either stories of the misunderstandings of local traditional culture on the part of the Western therapeutic agents or the local cultural resistance to the imposition of the implicit Western norms underpinning therapy (e.g. Brett, 1996; Ferraro, 2007, p. 399, Leach, 2015; Parker, 2014). The situation created by the rapid emergence of a new generation of therapists and clients in countries such India and China does not fit such templates and it will increasingly pose challenges to anyone assuming that the starting point for understanding psychotherapy transculturally remains that it is an intrinsically 'Western' practice. This will be the case both for the predictable defenders of established psychotherapeutic orthodoxies and their equally predictable relativist and postcolonial critics in equal measure.

Provincialising psychotherapy

Psychotherapy's status as a 'Western' discipline has been sustained by its greater influence in Europe and North America and the fact that the main centres of therapy training, research and clienteles have been in these areas, as much as it has been sustained by the triumphant narrative of a technology of Western origin whose destiny it was to 'conquer' the rest of the world. As this changes in the coming years, it raises the prospect that centres of power in the development of psychotherapy are about to become more globally dispersed. In this regard, psychotherapy will simply be treading a path that is also being followed by other 'cultural' industries, such as entertainment, media and academia. Dipesh Chakrabarty's (2000, p. 3) book, 'Provincializing Europe', referenced in the introduction to this collection, begins with a statement that the 'Europe' that he is referring to is not,

> the region of the world we call 'Europe'. That Europe, one could say, has already been provincialized by history itself.

Instead, it is the, 'imaginary figure' of a particular kind of, 'political modernity', based upon the ideals of the, 'European Enlightenment' that is Chakrabarty's (2000, p. 4) target of interrogation. His concern was that imaginary remains to be deconstructed as the ideal type underpinning political theory and practice, despite 'actual' Europe's growing historical provincialisation. It was as if the ideology of politics had yet to catch up with the actually changing social relations of global political economic power. Given the amount of attention that Chakrabarty pays in the book to deconstructing Marxism as an example of conventional Eurocentric Enlightenment thought, this perhaps constituted a rather ironically conventionally Marxist framing of the relationship between political economic relations and ideological superstructures. At any rate, the growing acceptance in Western politics and academia that the economic growth of India and China might mean accepting as equals political cultures that appear distinctly non-Enlightenment from European perspectives, such as Hindu nationalism or contemporary Chinese Communism, suggests that, in some regard at least, that ideology might be beginning to catch up with shifting political economic reality. Cambridge University Press' recent decision to censor large numbers of peer-reviewed articles considered subversive by the Chinese government may have been reversed. It does however offer us a glimpse of a likely future in which a shifting balance of global economic power exposes any previous consensus on when to acknowledge Enlightenment rights and when to deny them as the outcome of a particular historical moment that is now past. After all, the defence of Enlightenment values was always partial in practice, for example, as Chakrabarty (2000, p. 4) himself observes, the colonial moment preached those rights as abstract universal principles while denying them in legal and political practice to its colonised subjects. As China's economic power increasingly dwarves the UK's to simply view China's attempts to censor and Western academics' resistance to such attempts through the lens of 'colonialism' (as the Chinese authorities are happy to frame them) is to increasingly miss the point of the emergence of a multipolar world. If this is the case in academia, it is likely to equally be the case in psychotherapy as well, as Bangalore and Shanghai become as economically important to the development of theory and practice as Hampstead or Manhattan. Maybe Bose will be rediscovered from under Freud's shadow and maybe training curricula around the world will be rewritten in a manner that increasingly decentres the narrative of triumphant Western origin and conquest. Even if that history is not rewritten, the new texts and theories that are developed in the coming century will inevitably reflect this shifting influence in a manner that increasingly makes a model of Western cultural power hard to sustain.

A culture of manualisation and the manualisation of culture

The emergence of this new situation will see the development of new and enduring points of controversy and contention and many of these are high-lighted in this collection. One in particular, broadly speaking, is the continuation of a tension between standardised 'skill' and 'technique' driven approaches, often marked by increasingly detailed manuals or textbooks for training on the one hand, and more experiential intuitive approaches in which the teaching of such skills and techniques is seen more as a means by which a particular therapeutic sensibility and subjectivity is developed than as an end in and of itself. The title of one the texts that I was given in the first few weeks of my postgraduate psychotherapy training in Manchester, 'Two models of counsellor training: becoming a person or learning to be a skilled helper', (Jenkins, 1995) summed up the division as it presented itself to the course organisers. The first formulation comes from the title of Rogers (1961) famous collection of essays on humanistic person-centred psychotherapy and reflects the vision of a development of a particular caring and genuine relationship between therapist and client as the motor of the therapeutic change that was at the heart of his vision. Rogers makes clear the way in which he was influenced by a number of sources in the development of this model. One notable influence was the ambiguous influence of Freud, who provided some inspiration but was predominantly framed in negative terms as someone with a profoundly pessimistic view of human nature against which Rogers' more positive world-view could be expounded by contrast (although one of Freud's renegade disciples Otto Rank is simultaneously cited as a major positive influence). Here, Rogers can be seen as part of a long list of innovators in therapeutic theory of very different varieties, from Carl Jung up to Aaron Beck, all of whom had little choice (as we see in the case of the latter from *Rosner* in this collection) but to largely frame their new developments in terms of its departure from orthodox Freudianism. The other notable and more positive influence on Rogers was his religious world-view. He repeatedly references his Christian upbringing and beliefs as foundational, and the influence of Christian ideals such as that of universal love (*agape*) on elements of Rogers' philosophy such as the therapeutic ideal to be aimed for of the therapist holding the client in an attitude of 'unconditional positive regard' is clear. The influence of such religious beliefs on therapy and an understanding of where or whether a boundary line should be drawn between religious ways of seeing and being in the world and their therapeutic equivalents is an important issue reflected upon in two papers in this collection. The world of therapy today is more overtly 'culturally diverse' than in previous generations, both with the spread of therapy globally mentioned above on the one hand, and the more obviously culturally diverse populations that therapists working in nations such as the UK are likely to be dealing with on the other. One outcome of this is that issues regarding religious belief are more likely to be openly and open-mindedly addressed in training and they certainly came up with some regularity on the course that I trained on. Respecting (and indeed performing respect for) different religious beliefs has become a central component of how the trainee demonstrates her respect for cultural difference; an essential competence to be performed and audited in the new disciplinary regimes of therapeutic professionalisation. Valuable as this may be for those who wish religion to be shown the kind of respect that Freud was famously unwilling to show it, it still perhaps leaves us with the danger that religion is merely collapsed into culture and the uniquely religious aspects and sensibilities that matter to many practitioners become overlooked. This is a danger that has many parallels with the concern raised in *Harding's* article, that dialogues between religion and psychological therapies, can devolve into,

> the former simply serving the latter – as a provider of high-sounding, inspirational alternative terminologies for what is basically psychology, effectively masking a slide into agnosticism.

For some, such as *Harding*, maintaining a boundary between religious and other forms of experience and belief is an important piece of identity work to address. It is worth noting that for many therapeutic innovators whose 'religious' convictions were important to the development of their therapeutic sensibilities and techniques that the maintenance of this boundary did not appear to be such a concern however. *Harding* acknowledges that for Kosawa Heisaku, the main subject of *his* paper, 'the fruits of religion-psy dialogue emerged in two simple questions: what is insight, and what does it cost', neither of which seem to necessarily presuppose a strong interest in establishing and maintaining the boundaries between religious and psychological insight. The same would appear to be true of Rogers, the other main subject of *Harding's* paper. Rogers' main 'religious' inspiration was his Christianity but it does not appear to be the only 'religious' influence on the development of his thought. In an early example of cross-cultural influence in the development of therapeutic theory, Rogers (1961, p. 7) seems, by his own account, to have been much affected by a study visit to China whilst he was a university student and his writing on occasion mentions a 'Zen' or 'Daoist' ideal of flexibility and openness as the ideal end point of the self-actualised person that his school of therapy is intended to enable to come into being. Yet with Rogers there is similarly no sense that his religious inspirations are an essential or unique component of his therapeutic way of being to be distinguished from the other components of that way of being. The distinction between religious and psychological and/or cultural beliefs and ways of being might well indeed be important, but its importance can only really be addressed by first asking the question; 'important for who and in what context'?

The second formulation in the paper that I was given as a trainee, 'learning to be a skilled helper' may well be less familiar to many, being derived from the title of Egan's (1975/2010) 'Skilled Helper' model of therapy. In contrast to Rogers, Egan's model relies less on the development of a particular sensibility on the part of the therapist and more on the application of a series of steps designed to identify and isolate the client's problem and then develop strategies to address and solve it. First published in 1975, Egan's model can be seen as part of the trend towards the now omni-present and increasingly unquestionable manualisation of psychotherapy training and development mentioned in the introduction to this collection. It can also be seen as part of a zeitgeist that began a move away from the more holistic approach to personal development in the therapeutic relationship pioneered by Rogers and other humanists and existentialists in the immediate postwar years, towards a tendency to isolate problems or issues in the client's life to be addressed through the application of standardised problem solving techniques. This tendency is well encapsulated in *The Skilled Helper's* subtitle, 'a problem-management and opportunity-development approach to helping' As such it fitted the zeitgeist of other therapeutic development's, such as Becks' development of manualised CBT around the same time, described in *insert author*.

Despite the injunctions of our course leaders to develop our own individual therapeutic styles based upon our own combination of elements of previous theories, there was little doubt as to the direction that history was assumed to be taking. In the era of IAPT and similar government schemes to 'improve access' to therapy, then a move away from the Rogerian paradigm of personal development to the kind of skilled manualised training typified in different ways by Egan or Beck fits the zeitgeist for a number of reasons. It is measurable and quick, both to train and deliver. A therapist no longer requires her own lengthy and expensive personal therapy to qualify; the personal qualities of the therapist being secondary to her ability to demonstrate that she has acquired and is able to utilise the requisite check-list of skills. Likewise, it is quicker and cheaper to deliver, thereby 'improving access' (or a cynic might suggest 'hitting the targets').

By identifying and isolating specific problems that impair the 'functioning' of the client and resolving them quickly with her skills, as both Egan and Beck's (*see Rosner*) models encourage, the therapist is ideally able to return the client to work (and thereby improve her life) in a limited number of sessions, without the messy and often time-consuming work of personal exploration that marked earlier therapeutic regimes. As such, the move towards 'skilled helper' or CBT models dovetails in a very easy to understand manner with a particular regime of governance that aims to use therapy as a technology for the efficient, speedy and cost-effective production of healthy working citizens. One does not necessarily have to identify as either religious or secular to fear that something therapeutically invaluable is at risk of being lost in such a transition. As *insert author* observes, the introduction of 'Managed Healthcare Budgets' in the US dovetailed nicely with the rise of CBT for this reason, (whilst conversely being experienced by traditional psychoanalysts as an existential threat for precisely the same reasons (see Schechter, 2014). Similar processes lie behind the rapid rise to hegemony of CBT in state provided and funded services in the era of IAPT in the UK.

Marks notes the similarities between the development of 'rational therapy' in the Eastern bloc and the development of REBT and CBT and the latter's rise to dominance in the West. *Marks* rightly points to the importance of 'enlightenment ideals of rationality' in explaining this seemingly 'counterintuitive' similarity. Enlightenment rationality was however an ever-present feature of both Western and Soviet bloc culture throughout the twentieth century and the extent to which it underpinned (in a different manner) other therapeutic visions (not least Freud's). Perhaps an even more important linkage is the importance that both the Stalinist regimes of the East in the 1960s and 1970s and the neoliberal regimes of the 1980s onwards both, in their admittedly different ways, laid upon work and labour as a moral imperative. For governance regimes that seek to set and hit economic production targets (including for the production of economically productive subject-workers) then a therapeutic regime that mirrors that regime, with clear targets of progress to hit, both in terms of the progress of the individual client and the number of clients 'helped', fits perfectly. The rise of CBT in the era of IAPT would, in this regard, appear to be a part of far broader cultural trends.

Conclusions

It is in this context that contemporary moves to take 'culture' seriously within anthropology might need to be addressed. The need to de-centre some of the universalising assumptions of Western psychotherapies (such as Freud's) and the need to take seriously the unfamiliar aspects of the world-view and experience of clients from different backgrounds are important, and the move towards an appreciation of 'cultural' difference has been important on occasion in bringing these issues to the forefront of therapists' attention. It still remains important to look at the way that the idea of 'culture' is framed in such contemporary uses as itself being a particular kind of cultural artefact however, revealing of the conditions of its own production and circulation. 'Culture' is increasingly framed in professional regimes of training, accreditation and audit, such as therapy, as an object of expert knowledge, partially separate from the persons who are both its owners and outcome (e.g. Skeggs, 2004). In such a reified abstract form, it too can easily become another partially de-personalised item of skill and technique to add to the checklist. Rather than simply uncritically embracing therapy's current move towards understanding 'culture' as a long-overdue correction to its previous universalising tendency to the 'conquest' of different cultures, it might be wiser to take a more cautious approach that seeks to explore what aspects of the therapeutic experience the use of the concept illuminates *and* obscures in particular contexts. *Miller* points to the ways in which a particular vision of Scottish culture as a general entity and particularly its relationship to its English neighbour usefully enabled *him* to explore issues to do with national feelings of 'inferiority' that might otherwise not come to light. *He* is correct however to draw attention to the dangers that are also inherent in such an approach, such as over-generalisation and stereotyping. For the past thirty years, anthropology, the discipline that more than any other was responsible for developing the 'culture concept' in its current forms has increasingly moved away from such models of 'culture'. Instead anthropology has increasingly drawn attention to the ways in which in the idea of bounded homogenous cultures linked to particular bounded groups is made increasingly untenable by intensifying patterns of global interconnection (e.g. Appadurai, 1990). The discipline has also increasingly focused on the ways in which 'culture' as an idea is itself borne out of the need to make sense of particular experiences rather than being an inherent property of those experiences itself (e.g. Clifford, 1986). It would be a sad missing of the opportunity to rethink the relationship between culture and psyche as concepts if psychotherapy, along with similar professions, were to adopt that older model of understanding 'cultural difference' at precisely the moment when global cultural changes increasingly render it redundant.

Disclosure statement

No potential conflict of interest was reported by the author.

ORCID

Keir Martin ⓘ http://orcid.org/0000-0002-3157-0773

References

Akhtar, S., & Tummala-Narra, P. (2008). Psychoanalysis in India. In S. Akhtar (Ed.), *Freud along the Ganges: Psychoanalytic reflections on the people and culture of India* (pp. 3–25). New Delhi: Stanza.

Appadurai, A. (1990). Disjuncture and difference in the global cultural economy. *Theory, Culture and Society, 7*, 295–310.

Bose, G. (1949). The genesis and adjustment of the Oedipus myth. *Samiksa, 3*(1), 222–240.

Brett, E. (1996). The classification of posttraumatic stress disorder. In B. van der Kolk, A. McFarlane, & L. Weisath (Eds.), *Traumatic stress: The effects of overwhelming experience on mind, body, and society* (pp. 117–128). New York, NY: Guilford Press.

Chakrabarty, D. (2000). *Provincialising Europe: Postcolonial thought and historical difference.* Princeton: Princeton University Press.

Clifford, J. (Ed.). (1986). *Writing culture: The poetics and politics of ethnography.* Berkeley: University of California Press.

Egan, G. (2010[1975]). *The skilled helper: A problem-management and opportunity-development approach to helping.* Belmont: Brooks/Cole.

Ferraro, G. (2007). *Cultural anthropology: An applied perspective.* Belmont, CA: Thomson Wadworth.

Freehand, C. (2011). The rise of the new global elite. *The Atlantic.* Jan/Feb 2011 issue.

Herman, J. (1992). *Trauma and recovery.* New York, NY: Basic Books.

Huang, H.-Y. (2015, September). Therapy and the media in China. *Therapy Today*, pp. 8–11.

Hutz, C., & Gomes, W. (2013). Counseling and psychotherapy in Brazil: From private practice to community services. In R. Moodley, U. Gielen, & R. Wu (Eds.), *Handbook of counselling and psychotherapy in an international context* (pp. 95–105). New York, NY: Routledge.

Jenkins, P. (1995). Two models of counselor training: Becoming a person or learning to be a skilled helper. *Counselling, 6*(3), 203–206.

Kakar, S. (1978). *The inner world: A psychoanalytic study of childhood and society in India.* Oxford: Oxford University Press.

Kharas, H., & Gertz, G. (2010). The new global middle class: A crossover from West to East. In C. Li (Ed.), *China's emerging middle class: Beyond economic transformation.* Washington, DC: The Brookings Institution.

Kochlar, R., & Oates, R. (2015). *A global middle class is more promise than reality: From 2001 to 2011, nearly 700 million step out of poverty, but most only barely.* Washington, DC: Pew Research Center.

Leach, A. (2015, February 5). Exporting trauma: Can the talking cure do more harm than good? *The Guardian.*

Madsen, O. (2014). *The therapeutic turn: How psychology altered Western culture.* London: Routledge.

Matza, T. (2012). "Good individualism"? Psychology, ethics, and neoliberalism in postsocialist Russia. *American Ethnologist, 39*(4), 804–818.

Mauss, M. (1925/1966). *The gift: Forms and functions of exchange in archaic societies.* London: Cohen and West Limited.

Meckel, D. (2009). Hinduism and psychoanalysis. In J. Belzen (Ed.), *Changing the scientific study of religion: Beyond Freud?* (pp. 211–241). Dordrecht: Springer.

Moore, H. (2007). *The subject of anthropology: Gender, symbolism and psychoanalysis.* London: Polity.

Obeysekere, G. (1990). *The work of culture: Symbolic transformation in psychoanalysis and anthropology.* Chicago, IL: University of Chicago Press.

Parker, I. (2014). Foreword. In O. Madsen (Ed.), *The therapeutic turn: How psychology altered Western culture* (pp. vii–viii). London: Routledge.

Petty, J., & Bracken, P. (1998). *Rethinking the trauma of war.* London: Free Association Books.

Pezzini, M. (2012). *An emerging middle class.* OECD Observer. Retrieved February 1, 2017, from http://oecdobserver.org/news/fullstory.php/aid/3681/An_emerging_middle_class.html

Ramana, C. (1964). *On the early history and development of psychoanalysis in India.* Calcutta: Indian Psychoanalytical Society.

Rogers, C. (1961). *On becoming a person: A therapist's view of psychotherapy.* Boston, MA: Houghton Mifflin.

Schechter, K. (2014). *Illusions of a future: Psychoanalysis and the biopolitics of desire.* Durham, NC: Duke University Press.

Skeggs, B. (2004). *Class, self, culture.* London: Routledge.

Spiro, M. (1982). *Oedipus in the trobriands.* Chicago, IL: University of Chicago Press.

Young, A. (1995). *The harmony of illusions. Inventing post-traumatic stress disorder.* Princeton, NJ: Princeton University Press.

Zhang, L. (2016). The rise of therapeutic governing in postsocialist China. *Medical Anthropology, 35*(2), 119–131.

Therapy as cultural, politically influenced practice

Del Loewenthal

In order to look at how National Institute for Health and Care Excellence (NICE) in the UK attempts to measure psychotherapeutic work it is argued that it is necessary to first consider the nature of psychotherapeutic knowledge. Hence, this article is divided into four parts. The first is looking at the psychological therapies (and research) as cultural practices, the second is the workings of NICE in relation to psychotherapy, the third is looking at what may be the changes in our society that have given rise to the current prevalence of cognitive behaviour therapy (CBT), and the fourth is what, if anything, can be done? It is argued that regarding mental health psychiatry and psychology are based on false foundations, and unfortunately our governments seem determined that psychotherapy should follow suit.

Is it now the case that the psychological therapies in the United Kingdom (UK), far more than psychiatry and psychology, are being asked to comply with an evidence-based practice that has been constructed to favour approaches which do not enable clients and patients to explore meaning in-depth? It will be argued that a revolution has already started whereby freedom as to what is carried out by psychological therapists and explored by their clients has, as with so many areas of our lives, become severely restricted. It would appear that psychological therapists' professional bodies attempt to go along with this audit culture and pseudo-science, desperately trying to get their modalities accepted. It will be argued that the result is that the psychological therapies have lost their way in unwittingly becoming agents of the state. This process has greatly reduced not only the choice that is being offered to patients and clients, but reduces the extent to which the psychological therapies can be essentially subversive and can provide a confidential space where clients have the freedom to explore anything that comes to their minds. An illustration of how such changes come about is explored through how National Institute for Health and Care Excellence (NICE) attempts to measure the effects of psychotherapy. However, in contrast to the audit culture of New Public Management (Barzelay 2001; Gruening 2001) what will first be looked at here is the nature of psychotherapeutic work which psychotherapists seem in danger of forgetting, before examining how its erroneous measurement is catastrophically changing what was originally thought of as the psychotherapeutic project. It will be argued that at least in the UK, psychotherapists are in a war and there may just be a chance we could wake up and do something before it is too late. This article is in four sections: The first is looking at the psychological therapies (and research) as cultural practices; the second is the workings of NICE in relation to psychotherapy; the third is looking at what may be the changes in our society that have given rise to the current prevalence of cognitive behavioural therapy (CBT); and the fourth is what, if anything, can be done? The concern is that with regard to mental health, psychiatry and psychology are based on false foundations, and unfortunately UK governments seem determined that psychotherapy should follow suit.

It can be argued that what Freud, Klein, and others developed were practices. Whilst these practices evolved from others theorising previous practices, Freud, Klein, and others devised further theories (now over 600 of them (ref)) to explain these new practices. More recently, certain types of research have been the order of the day in order to justify these theories. Isn't it a mistake to look at the relation of theory and practice in psychotherapy, psychoanalysis, counselling, and the arts and play therapies (which are collectively referred to here as the 'psychological therapies') in terms of theories supplying the foundational underpinnings of practices? Thus, the associated theories, whilst they can be helpful, are not foundational and that perhaps to consider them as such might even be seen as delusional! Isn't it possible for a theory to have implications but to consider any theory, individually or collectively, as the foundation or as an application, as might particularly be seen in cases of manualisation, is based on a false premise? Several questions will therefore be raised:

1. Are the psychological therapies first and foremost practices?
2. Are theories attempts to explain practice or is theory the basis of our practice?
3. Do changes in this practice have more to do with changes in our culture that lead us to be more interested in different theories?
4. What are the forces in our society that make CBT so prevalent to the extent that such notions in our case of using randomised controlled trials (RCTs) as a so-called evidence based are used for the state-sanctioning of therapeutic practice?
    This last question is of particular importance and is connected with:
5. To what extent are psychiatry and psychology in the UK primarily agents of the state and is this now also happening to the psychological therapies?

There are, however, many further questions which we might ask about our practice, regardless of whether it is called CBT. CBT can be helpful, but as with other approaches, cannot be the only game in town. For example, what place if any in the psychological therapies have:

1. The medical model?
2. The DSM?
3. Psychoanalysis?
4. Science?
5. Also, to what extent is our attachment to a particular theory/theories to do with inadequacies in our own foundations and to what extent does any change appear to threaten our very foundations?

So, is the questioning of CBT just a part of a process of denial from some psychological therapists who aren't in the ascendancy and are taking it out on the state? Are all these different psychotherapeutic notions really to keep the psychotherapist occupied while something else therapeutically useful can happen? Can any modality really claim to be the only game in town?

There is the question whether in this context psychological therapists can actually diagnose and treat as in the medical model. But if I break my heart as opposed to breaking a limb can anyone, let alone a technician, tell me what my desire should be? NICE's work with regard to physical medicine is not be questioned here. They have done excellent work in attempting to get drug companies to report all their RCTs rather than just the successful ones, which perhaps shows what it is possible to get away with when using the term 'RCT.' Yet using RCTs for mental health can be regarded as misplaced. Not only is the theorising scandalous, as my colleague James Davies (2013) amongst others has shown, but any psychotropic medication is only required to be tested once after eight weeks, yet what of the people who are on it for more than eight weeks and in too many cases the rest of their lives? We have Richard Layard (2005) to thank for getting successive governments to accept the use of talking therapies over drug therapies. So what also of our own classification of different modalities? Can any be scientifically proven to be better than another? Yet Cotton in his research showed that others, who also had a psychiatric diagnosis, needed for their recovery therapeutic relationships where they could explore personal meaning (Cotton and Loewenthal 2015). But where is such research in State provision and policing of the psychological therapies?

Psychological therapies as cultural practices

The case is being made here for the place of practice at the heart of psychotherapy and counselling (Loewethal 2011). This primacy of practice can be seen as dating back to the time of Pyrrhonian scepticism to, more recently, the writings of Wittgenstein (1958), where what we do can be understood to be more about the activities in which we participate with our clients. There is therefore an increasing body of opinion showing the futility of theory as the basis of the psychological therapies (Brown and Stenner 2009; Frie and Orange 2009; Heaton 2013) and, with it, what is currently regarded as research. But the psychological therapies are also cultural practices, an attempt is being made here to reformulate an understanding of meaning as contextual and emerging through meeting of psychological therapist and client.

Thus, how we understand such emerging meaning will be mediated by cultural practices through the mixture of ideas that permeate our society in any period. Therefore, an attempt is being made here to describe a potential cultural movement that currently pervades and in some ways pragmatically and strategically, CBT so helpfully meets for some. However, with regard to false foundations it is not only CBT, but any therapies whether they be humanistic, existential, or psychoanalytic, which become totalising approaches, are potentially violent. At best, such theories are secondary; whilst they may have implications they can never provide a foundation to the primacy of practice.

Psychotherapists are involved with such aspects as talk, ritual, and gesture as in any meeting. Yet one does not do it based on theory, it is a practice, a cultural practice which can change within a culture and can be different between cultures, as the contributors to this book show. If one theorises about practice, it is done outside of practice; it is different. Also, one might end up theorising about the bone and muscle properties of the hand and arm or even the mouth as one speaks and gestures but it won't help much.

Isn't it the same with all psychological therapies – they involve something other than theoretical knowledge? Also, isn't much of psychology unhelpful here – learning about the ear or the larynx doesn't usually help us as psychotherapists? Are counselling and psychotherapeutic theories any better? Does Bion (1965) come closest to theorising practice with his system 'O' (the ineffable: the unknowable or ultimate truth)? Or is Polyani (1966) better with his notion of tacit knowledge? There again to what extent is well-being or the good to do with the knowledge derived from research?

How are we with patients/clients might be seen as an act of judgment and we might reflect on what we have said but does that make us practitioner researchers? Not if we take research to mean achieving generalisation through some systematic approach.

Research as a cultural practice

Psychotherapy as a cultural practice has, or attempts to, obtained legitimacy through whatever is taken as the means to do this for that particular cultural time. Often these days empirical research is the legitimising tool and this more recently has to be 'evidence based' without having to consider what is the evidence of, for example, love or intimacy. Is research another cultural practice? As one person who took part in a significant RCT said when I asked what her research had to do with truth and justice, 'Not much' she said, 'but I got my modality accepted.' (We then of course get researcher allegiance to boot.)

Research is what all psychotherapeutic professional bodies are pushing us to do. Yet isn't this another cultural practice that is linked to legitimising changes in our culture? How can anyone with a grade C or above in Maths GCSE ever claim that RCTs could be the gold standard for so much psychotherapy research? Indeed, through the work that I was commissioned to do by United Kingdom Council for Psychotherapy (UKCP), which also appeared as 'Scrutinising NICE' (see Guy et al. 2012), questions were asked in the House. Subsequently such fundamental flaws were acknowledged by the previous and current head of NICE, and there was a desperate attempt to find another method whereby our modalities can be objectively evaluated whilst RCTs looked set to only continue temporarily as the order of the day. What research is really then of use to psychotherapeutic practitioners? It is argued here very little if we think in terms of generalisation. Indeed for those interested in research it seems the most important aspect of psychotherapeutic work is to remind people how the consequences of attempting to apply so-called evidence-based research findings may be more detrimental than beneficial. Isn't Physis or Phusis what comes out if its self? But now the measuring instruments determine the therapy, and as Vygotsky (1962) states we are all shaped by the tools and instruments we come to use.

There is a changing fashion in what is regarded as research – what was acceptable as a doctorate some years ago can be different to what is acceptable in the same discipline today, where empirical, positivistic research in psychotherapy is in the ascendancy. Theoretical explorations are rarely now considered by our professional bodies as research or indeed by an increasing number of university departments where one will be lucky if it is classified instead by what is regarded as the less significant term 'scholarship.' Now quantitative empirical studies rule the day in psychotherapy.

What has research got to do with thoughtful practice? I have been interested in different types of research and was indeed the Chair of UKCP's first Research Committee, but I regard most of what is now research in the psychological therapies, whether it be quantitative or qualitative, as being of little value. Indeed as Merleau-Ponty (1962) has said sometimes if one attempts to take away the mystery one can take away the thing itself. Or to put it another way, as happened when a French Minster of Health, Philippe Douste-Blazy, was under pressure to evaluate psychoanalysis and replied: 'Psychoanalysis is something else and we should let it be' (Snell 2007).

I have previously used the name 'post-existentialism' to tentatively being put forward in an attempt to describe a potential cultural moment whereby the psychological therapies can be considered to at least start with practice and counter the hegemony of training technicians as psychological therapists perhaps to oil the wheels of our increasingly dominant managerialist culture (see, for example, Loewenthal 2010).

Whatever the name, is it possible to have an approach to the psychological therapies which attempts to enable individuals to experience their alienation in the hope that they may still be able, individually and collectively, to do more about it? When I was a student we all read and talked about alienation. Now we seem to be so alienated that this is no longer possible. With the psychological therapies aren't we meant to open a space up where people, if they want to, can confidentially explore any thought, dream, fantasy, or problem with others, including those in authority? Indeed shouldn't the psychological therapies be essentially subversive if they are to be potentially free of existing power structures? Is it really inevitable for governments to have the power to decide whether to endorse us to allow clients/patients to explore meanings in their specific contexts, without ignoring the work of the post-modernists, the psychoanalysts, or the political? Or was that just about ok previously for a few but when there are now over 1 million people per year in this country having therapy (Chunn 2013) are previous freedoms now too great a risk in terms of social control? Is that why the extraordinary recent interest in the provision and controlling of the psychological therapies?

Can we finally get rid of RCTs?

Don't we already have our own way of being thoughtful about our work in, for example, taking it to clinical supervision and writing and presenting papers? Arguments regarding the inappropriateness of RCTs in the psychological therapies can be found elsewhere (for example, House and Loewenthal 2008).

NICE work if you can get it: Can you get how NICE works?

Whilst there is also the question that perhaps 'it's not such nice work even if you can get it!' However, I was hoping some people might also read this as 'Can you get how NICE works?'

In 'Scrutinising NICE' (Guy et al. 2012) we provided the following overview:

- Consequences for patient choice of NICE guidelines implemented via Improving Access to Psychological Therapies (IAPT).
- NICE's methodology has been inappropriately applied to the talking therapies.
- The relevance of the assumptions which underpin NICE's preferred research method, RCTs, is questioned.
- Whilst NICE recognises many of the issues raised concerning its methodology, it is *acting* as though they don't exist.
- The case is examined that the current process works in favour of some therapies (e.g. CBT) and puts others at an unreasonable disadvantage.
- NICE should adopt a pluralist approach to research methodologies, following the lead of the American Psychological Association (APA).

It would appear that successive heads of NICE recognise the inappropriateness of RCTs but don't know what to replace this with. For those not familiar with the process for the NICE, we think it is important that you note their language. It is embedded in a model of biological medicine where patients' experiences (*symptoms*) are indicative of underlying *conditions* which need to be *diagnosed* in order for an appropriate *treatment* to be *prescribed* (a language which I imagine a few people warm to and others don't). What happens is as follows:

- A '**condition**' on which to issue guidelines about **treatment options is selected.**
- A '**Guideline Development Group**' (GDG) is created.
- Research conducted on 'interventions' for participants who have been '**diagnosed**' with the '**condition**' giving primacy to those studies which have used RCTs is examined.

NICE does seem to recognise concerns about such constructions of depression as a clinical condition, but all their guidelines are based on evidence gathered around patients who have been diagnosed with a relevant condition – as Bentall (2009) points out, such diagnostic systems have no evidence of usefulness.

Regarding NICE's GDGs 'the exact composition of the GDG should be tailored to the topic covered by the clinical guideline. It should reflect the range of stakeholders and groups whose professional activities or care will be covered by the guidelines' (NICE 2009:29). One of the problems here is that if stakeholders do not recognise the use of diagnoses then their 'research evidence' is not included. Some psychoanalytic schools do use diagnoses in a more metaphorical use of the medical model. 'The person's individuality eventually becomes more impressive than his or her conformity with an abstraction'. However, a significant number of psychotherapists, researchers, and doctors do not believe diagnoses of mental health conditions are valid. With regard to psychiatry the psychiatrist Middleton (2015), "Fully realised, these criticisms of the evidence supporting professionalised mental health services and practices have profound implications. At face value they can be read *'There is no conclusive science supporting claims that any of the psycho-pharmaceuticals work as claimed, and when they do help, it is as likely as not that "help" is the result of complex phenomena not indistinguishable from placebo'* and *'Useful outcomes of a psychological therapy are primarily the result of a helpful relationship, rather than the result of any identifiable psychotherapeutic technique'* (p. 29). If these conclusions were to be widely acknowledged, then much of what conventional mental health services are commissioned to do would have to be seen as acts of faith rather than fact. In the event few have reacted to *Beyond the Current Paradigm* (ref) with any rebuttal of these underpinning conclusions, despite the fact that it was published in the house magazine of the Royal College of Psychiatrists."

But back to NICE. NICE does seem to be, on the one hand, aware of some of the problems; so, for example, it is stated that their GDG for Depression *"considered it important to acknowledge the uncertainty inherent in our current understanding of depression and its classification, and that assuming a false categorical certainty is likely to be unhelpful and, even worse, damaging*" (NICE 2009:23–24). However, despite these factors, NICE only seriously considered research evidence conducted using participants with depression as a firm 'diagnosis' (e.g. NICE 2009:262).

So who in fact makes up the stakeholders in these GDGs who play an essential part in NICE's recommendations, which includes 'where evidence is lacking the guidelines incorporate statements and recommendations based upon consolidated statements developed by the GDG' (NICE 2009:12). The GDG for Depression comprises Chair: Consultant Psychiatrist, Psychiatrists: 2; Psychological Therapist: 1; Psychotherapist: 1; Clinical Psychologists: 2; GPs: 2; Nurses: 2; Pharmacist: 1; Service Users: 2; Carer: 1 (15 in total including Chair).

This can lead to groups with strong vested interests: in fact at the time of publishing our work on 'Scrutinising NICE' (Guy et al. 2012), and unfortunately little seems to be changed subsequently, an overall review of the composition of the GDGs producing the clinical guidelines on anxiety, depression in adults, and schizophrenia showed 6.7% were psychological therapists and 33% from the medical profession. Furthermore, 36% were from the National Collaborating Centre for Mental Health. And who are they? They are 'a partnership between the Royal College of Psychiatry and the British Psychological Society's Centre for Outcome Research and Effectiveness' (NICE 2009:13) whose director is a clinical psychologist. You might say 'at least we have a psychotherapist and a psychological therapist on the GDG for Depression to attempt to counterbalance this.' Though what is the distinction between psychotherapist and psychological therapist? But let's see who they are: one is a Consultant Cognitive Behavioural Psychotherapist, and the other 'holds psychodynamic psychotherapy and supervision qualifications' and also happens to be the Chair of the New Savoy Partnership, a government-funded body whose aim is to implement nationally IAPT 'evidence-based practice.' It could be argued that there is not a balanced representation of psychological therapists given that at this particular time the representation is only through the Chair of the New Savoy Partnership (an organisation designed to promote IAPT) and a Consultant Cognitive Behavioural Psychotherapist, and those clinical psychologists from the National Collaborating Centre for Mental Health who are 'committed to CBT-type research closely involved in developing NICE guidelines' (Mollon 2009). Yet psychological therapists appear to have been regarded as one homogenous professional group. It *matters* that NICE appears not to have ensured adequate representation of psychotherapists.

"*Where evidence is lacking, the guidelines incorporate statements and recommendations based upon the consensus statements developed by the GDG*" (NICE, 2009:12).

Again, NICE appears to state some of the limitations but doesn't act on it. For example, "*the importance of organising care in order to support and encourage a good therapeutic relationship is at times as important as the specific treatments offered*" (NICE, 2009:12–13).

"It is difficult to determine whether or not the benefits ... resulted specifically from the therapy or the prolonged contact with the therapist during that time" (NICE, 2009:162).

"The quality of the relationship consistently predicts outcome, independent of the espoused model or condition being treated" Pilgrim et al. (2009:244). So how come the so-called gold standard research method, RCTs, is precisely one that attempts to neutralise the effect of a particular therapist?

What has really led to the current prevalence of CBT?

Wouldn't it be good if there were more people in government like that previously mentioned by French Minister of Health, Philippe Douste-Blazy, who stated 'psychic suffering is neither measurable nor open to evaluation' (Snell 2007). In this review Snell also writes,

> For where the British psychoanalytic establishment has, for the most part, been anxious to go along with the challenge to produce 'evidence' and demonstrate 'treatment efficacy,' the francophone world – as represented here, at least – will have none of it. In ... the book, Yves Cartuyvels, an eminent Belgian professor of law who has spent his professional life examining the nature of evidence, refutes the claims of cognitive-behavioural therapy to be founded – 'objectively' and 'scientifically' – in solid evidence. Such claims are mere scientism; they rest on 'a superannuated conception of science as the measure of ultimate truth' and a naïve nineteenth-century scientific positivism: 'the epistemology of science might as well not have bothered underlining, as it has been doing for many years, the social construction of science, or describing the interplay of its actors, and the interests and values behind the practice of science.' These claims also necessitate a refusal to accept that a patient might choose 'a rationality other than scientific rationality in response to psychic malaise.' In any case what, Cartuyvels asks, is 'effective' in the field of mental health? 'The suppression of a symptom? Help with living with a symptom? Who fixes and defines the thresholds of effectiveness? Science? The therapist? The subject? Are these thresholds the same from one individual to another, from one kind of suffering to another?'. (Snell 2007)

In concluding our previous research on 'Scrutinising NICE' (2012) we summarised that whilst NICE recognises many of the issues concerning its methodology, it ends up acting as if they don't exist.

It would appear that NICE decided that a review was not required. This is despite UKCP working with others, including the British Psychoanalytic Council (BPC), the Psychotherapists from the Royal College of Psychiatrists, British Association for Counselling and Psychotherapy (BACP), and Association of Child Psychotherapists (ACP), submitting a joint consultation response on NICE's guideline manual. For many the consequences are that patient choice is greatly reduced and there is likely to be decreasing work opportunities for psychological therapists who are not accredited to use sanctioned, evidence-based modalities. So how has this come about and what if anything can be done?

This is now considered, drawing on *Critical Psychotherapy, Psychoanalysis and Counselling: Implications for Practice* (Loewenthal 2015). The prevailing climate appears to facilitate the growth of manualised, state-regulated therapies, aimed at taking clients' minds off their concerns and delivered by 'technicians' (Mace et al. 2009; Parker & Revelli 2008). As one IAPT evaluator has put it, there has been a transformation in practice in recent years, moving from a 'cottage industry to a factory-based production line' (Parry et al. 2010) with equally disruptive effects for practitioners. Perhaps we should consider our modality, whatever it is, and wonder about the use of, often so-called, 'science' in the pursuit of vested interests' notions of progress and authority.

In an era where through Edward Snowden's revelations our telephone calls and emails are monitored in the name of internal security, there would appear to have been a significant shift from accepting talking therapies as essentially both confidential and subversive, and inevitably being located on the edges of our society. However, with practices and trainings becoming *increasingly* registered, regulated, and incorporated into mainstream society, the result is the constant risk assessment of this confidentiality (Loewenthal 2014). An increasingly pervasive audit culture and limited notions of evidence-based practice, involving some dubious claims to be 'scientific,' can be seen as legitimising this change. Yet isn't this more to do with the attempts of those in power at a particular time to determine what is and is not science? As Foucault states, '…if we ask what is, in its very general form, the kind of division governing our will to knowledge – then we may well discern something like a system of exclusion (historical, modifiable, institutionally constraining)' (Foucault 1971).

Our students, at least in the UK, are increasingly seeing their training as a commodity they are purchasing as customers rather than as a personal exploration. A concern here was, and still is, once critical psychotherapy, psychoanalysis, and counselling is established it will become a minority module on mainstream programmes. The implication therefore is that it will become by definition primarily 'uncritical,' but the 'critical' add-on will allow for a notion of democracy, and perhaps what is becoming an illusion of academic freedom. What is new, however, is the increasing extent of the state's involvement in purchasing/providing specific psychological therapies, alongside our new era of neoliberalism and the New Public Management (Barzelay 2001; Gruening 2001) with its audit culture and its 'Markets, Managers and Measurement.'

There seem to be two parallel developments taking place in the talking therapies in the UK. First, we have neoliberalism which encourages 'the privatisation of everything public and the commercialisation of all things private' (Barber 2000). This affects our relationships (Verhaeghe 2014), including what is meant by the notion of public service and how we attempt to educate. It can be argued that the introduction of 'New Public Management' provides a smokescreen for such privatisation. However, in the name of safeguarding the public, the state is simultaneously tightening its grip on the psychological therapies. Certainly there have been some abuses by psychotherapists as well as doctors, nurses, and other professionals, but isn't there now far more managerial abuse with far fewer checks and balances than previously?

Verhaeghe (2014) has argued that neoliberalism has brought out the worst in us, in which case where does psychotherapy, psychoanalysis, and counselling place itself, if it can, in relation to these cultural changes? Can 'critical' psychotherapy, psychoanalysis, and counselling provide an alternative space within this neoliberal culture where the talking therapies are increasingly becoming agents of social control? Or will the talking therapies only be allowed to survive if we don't rock the neoliberalist boat too much? The market that was supposed to emancipate us appears instead to have offered atomisation and loneliness. So what of 'the common good' in both this and our work as talking therapists? Furthermore, whilst we as talking therapists see people whose work is alienating and mainly offers extrinsic rewards, isn't even our own work becoming one where '[t]he workplace has been overwhelmed by a mad, Kafkaesque infrastructure of assessments, monitoring, measuring, surveillance and audits, centrally directed and rigidly planned....' (Monbiot 2014). It would also appear that if too many people understand a particular audit process it has to be changed!

The Layard report (2005) and the recommendations for the talking therapies from the NICE (2009) have possibly had the greatest effect on psychotherapy, psychoanalysis, and counselling in the UK. First, the Layard report has been influential in that it has convinced successive governments in putting the case for the talking therapies in contrast to pharmaceutical interventions. Second, governments are increasingly taking mental health needs seriously. The IAPT national programme provides for mental health on a population-based basis, and so the government's role becomes central to the training, provision, and delivery of talking therapy. This results in a focus on what many see as narrowly defined evidence-based practices (where, for example, is their evidence for intimacy and love?). Favoured approaches tend to meet the imposed measurement systems; these seem to be those approaches that take clients' minds off their problems rather than attempting to help them work through what is bothering them. These favoured approaches are those talking therapies where the evidence base has been established through RCTs, and the public are encouraged to seek these out. Yet RCTs can be seen to be, at best, highly questionable as a way of investigating therapeutic approaches (Dalal 2019; Guy et al. 2012). We can hopefully only imagine the incredulity of future generations, given the questions over how appropriate, if not scientifically absurd, RCTs are for investigating any therapeutic approach, including those that are manualised (Guy et al. 2012). Perhaps much of CBT's popularity is due to how we both individually, and through the state and other interested parties attempt to dilute both our own sexuality and violence and conspire not to step outside the ideology that contains us.

In the talking therapies there was the idea that patients/clients could explore what they found problematic in being clear about themselves. Often, what needed to be spoken about was taboo within the particular culture they came from. However, as a result of the involvement of the State in the talking therapies there is an increasing possibility that patients/clients cannot now speak of what is not usually permissible or taboo. There is also the possibility that trainings do not sufficiently equip talking therapists to hear what is usually not said, and to be able to stay with not knowing.

One conclusion I drew in the book *Critical Psychotherapy, Psychoanalysis and Counselling: Implications for Practice* (Loewenthal 2015) is that three very difficult personal and collective courses of action may be required if we are able to significantly change our practices: The first is Plato's plea (Cushman 2002) that Therapiea is about continuing to remind ourselves and others that whilst science and technology are important, they should always come second to the resources of the human soul. Second, we are all capable of good and evil and we therefore need to be aware of those theories that encourage us to sidestep any consideration of our capability for making others wretched. Third, as individuals we wish to escape through denial, unsavoury aspects of ourselves, and so can therefore be seduced or otherwise forced away from really opening up to both ourselves and our clients/patients. This is facilitated by the powers-that-be, which in our case is neoliberalist capitalism (Verhaeghe 2014). Yet the assumption remains that the more we can stay open to all this and work it through, then the greater ours and others' potentiality.

There is much to support the idea that the state is using psychotherapy, psychoanalysis, and counselling as a form of social control. Although it can be argued that oppressing oppresses the oppressor, perhaps it is particularly pertinent that in some ways don't both oppressors and oppressed wish to be oppressed? Perhaps we welcome this 'opportunity'; although both Marx and Nietzsche have suggested in different ways that religion enables people to stop thinking, the demise of religion for some would appear to have been replaced by the forces of both consumerism and the state, which have resulted in the development of alienated states of being. For example, state-endorsed therapies tend to provide either a way of directly taking one's mind off what worries one (CBT), or a means of reflecting back that we are the persons that we would like to think of ourselves as; or, to a decreasing extent, approaches that do neither. What are almost too difficult to find are therapies that allow us to acknowledge the good in ourselves and others without denying our sexuality and violence, as well as a place in which we can consider our part in the political set-up.

Given the contributions in this volume what, if anything, can be done?

So what seems to be clear is that the talking therapies are cultural practices and the ways in which they are researched are also cultural practices. How should one respond to the inappropriateness of forcing an external empirical research method onto psychotherapy, psychoanalysis, and counselling? As Ricoeur (1970) writes, the hermeneutics of suspicion are in opposition to scientific understanding such that, for example, one should not attempt to locate psychoanalysis within the causal discourse of natural sciences which

Freud also attempted and is currently increasingly prevalent. However, qualitative research is often not much of an answer. Although it may help an individual researcher it cannot usually be generalised, and indeed shouldn't. Given that the notion of the practitioner researcher (McLeod 1999) means that increasingly trainees are probably worse than wasting their time with regard to preparing for their practice, it may be preferable for these students to consider social, economic, and technological contexts, or literary studies, instead of learning about statistics and a bit of biology. Taking bright people with the desire to help others and filling their minds with substandard technical thinking can be seen as another form of social control. Furthermore, as Rizq (2013) writes, the work of the talking therapist is increasingly becoming detrimental to the therapist's own life as well.

And as for the future training of psychotherapists could it become more like the training of psychiatrists and psychologists, making those who originally wanted to help others instead be caught up in state-endorsed frameworks.

In concluding the book on critical psychotherapy (Loewenthal 2015) what emerged were two key forces. The first is from the individual who, through what some would call denial, wants to avoid staying with uncomfortable thoughts, fantasies, and dreams. The second force is from those who do not want those that they manage to understand how this is done.

I fear that unless we as psychological therapists can re-establish the place we take up in contemporary society then we are rapidly, with regard to individual alienation and wretchedness, becoming far too much the problem rather than the solution.

In conclusion as my co-editor, Sonu Shamdasani states earlier:

> In recent years, a small but significant body of work has arisen studying histories of psychotherapies in discrete local contexts throughout the world, which is expanding and reframing our knowledge of them. However, little has been done to draw this work together within a comparative setting, and to chart the intersection of these connected histories and transcultural networks of exchange of knowledge and healing practices.

This book then has Shamdasani and his international colleagues work together with the two respondents making up the preceding chapters. To this has been added in this chapter my own interests in considering the psychological therapies as cultural rather than evidence-based practices. For here, it has also argued that current psychotherapeutic research studies, including 'evidence-based,' are again cultural practices such that science is misused to back up rather than lead change brought about by other forces in our societies. It is hoped therefore that such explorations of transcultural histories of psychotherapies also provide further weight to question others successful attempts for practitioners to blindly wrongly accept the concept of evidence-based practice (amongst many others) as if it were a value-free universal science. Hence, questioning 'evidence based' is just one of many implications from this research describing different cultural histories and addressing methodologically issues in carrying out a comparative history on these stories amongst stories.

References

Barber, B. (2000) 'Ballots versus Bullets' *Financial Times* 20th October 2000.

Barzelay, M. (2001) *The New Public Management: Improving Research and Policy Dialogue* Berkeley, Los Angeles, London: University of California Press.

Bentall, R. (2009) Guardian.co.uk 31 August 2009 [Online] Retrieved from: www. guardian.co.uk/commentisfree/2009/aug/31/psychiatry-psychosis-schizophrenia-drug-treatments.

Bion, W. (1965) *Transformations* London: Heinemann.

Brown, S. and Stenner, P. (2009) *Psychology without Foundations: History, Philosophy and Psychosocial Theory* London: Sage.

Chunn, L. (2013) 'Britain on the Couch: UK Therapists Share our Biggest Worries' *The Guardian* 7th December 2013.

Cotton, T. and Loewenthal, D. (2015) 'Personal versus Medical Meanings in Breakdown, Treatment and Recovery from "Schizophrenia"' *In:* Loewenthal, D. (ed) *Critical Psychotherapy, Psychoanalysis and Counselling: Implications for Practice*, Basingstoke: Palgrave Macmillan, pp. 77–92.

Cushman, R. (2002) *Therapeia: Plato's Conception of Philosophy* New Brunswick and London: Transaction Publishers.

Dalal, F. (2019) *CBT – The Cognitive Behavioural Tsunami: Managerialism, Politics and the Corruption of Science* Abingdon: Routledge.

Davies, J. (2013) *Cracked: Why Psychiatry is Doing More Harm than Good* London: Icon Books.

Foucault, M. (1971) 'The Discourse on Language' (trans. Swyre, R.) *Social Science Information* April 7–30.

Frie, R. and Orange, D. (Eds). (2009) *Beyond Postmodernism: New Dimensions in Clinical Theory and Practice* New York: Routledge.

Gruening, G. (2001) 'Origin and Theoretical Basis of New Public Management' *International Public Management Journal* 4.1–25.

Guy, A., Loewenthal, D., Thomas, R. and Stephenson, S. (2012) 'Scrutinising NICE: The Impact of the National Institute for Health and Clinical Excellence Guidelines on the Provision of Counselling and Psychotherapy in Primary Care in the UK' *Psychodynamic Practice*, 18, 1.

Heaton, J.M. (2013) *The Talking Cure: Wittgenstein on Language as Bewitchment and Clarity* Basingstoke: Palgrave Macmillan.

House, R. and Loewenthal, D. (Eds). (2008) *Against and for CBT: Towards a Constructive Dialogue?* Ross-on-Wye: PCCS Books.

Layard, R. (2005) 'Mental Health: Britain's Biggest Social Problem?' Paper presented at the No. 10 Strategy Unit Seminar on Mental Health, LSE 20th January 2005. Available at: www.cep.lse.ac.uk/textonly/research/mentalhealth/RL414d.pdf Accessed: December 31st 2012.

Loewenthal, D. (2010) 'Audit, Audit Culture and *Therapeia*: Some implications for Wellbeing with Particular Reference to Children' *In:* King, L. and Moutsou, C. (eds) *Rethinking Audit Cultures: A Critical Look at Evidence Based Practice in Psychotherapy and Beyond*, Ross-on-Wye: PCCS Books, pp. 75–95.

Loewenthal, D. (2011) *Post-Existentialism and the Psychological Therapies: Towards a Therapy without Foundations* London: Karnac.

Loewenthal, D. (2014) 'Are psychological Therapists Less Trustworthy than they used to be?' *European Journal of Psychotherapy & Counselling*, 16:2, 97–100.

Loewenthal, D. (Ed). (2015) *Critical Psychotherapy, Psychoanalysis and Counselling: Implications for Practice* Basingstoke: Palgrave Macmillan.

Mace, C., Rowland, N., Evans, C., Schroder, T. and Halstead, J. (2009) 'Psychotherapy Professionals in Europe: Expansion and Experiment' *European Journal of Psychotherapy & Counselling*, 11:2, 131–140.

McLeod, J. (1999) *Practitioner Research in Counselling* London: Sage.

Merleau-Ponty, M. (1962) *The Phenomenology of Perception* London: Routledge.

Middleton, H. (2015) 'The Medical Model: What Is It, Where Did It Come from and how Long Has It Got?' *In:* Loewenthal, D. (ed) *Critical Psychotherapy, Psychoanalysis and Counselling: Implications for Practice*, Basingstoke: Palgrave Macmillan, pp. 29–40.

Mollon, P. (2009) 'The NICE Guidelines are Misleading, Unscientific and Potentially Impede Good Psychological Care and Help' *Psychodynamic Practice* 15:1, 9–24.

Monbiot, G. (2014) 'Sick of this Market-driven World? You Should Be' *The Guardian* 5th August 2014.

NICE (2009) 'Treatment and Management of Depression in Adults (CG90). National Collaborating Centre for Mental Health' Published by The British Psychological Society 2010 [Online]. Available at: www.guidance.nice.org.uk/CG90/Guidance/pdf/English.

Parker, I. and Revelli, S. (2008) *Psychoanalytic Practice and State Regulation* London: Karnac.

Parry, G., Blackmore, C., Beecroft, C. and Booth, A. (2010) *A Systematic Review of the Efficacy and Clinical Effectiveness of Group Analysis and Analytic/ Dynamic Group Psychotherapy* Available at: www.academia.edu/2723418/A_systematic_review_of_the_efficacy_and_clinical_effectiveness_of_group_analysis_and_analytic_and_dynamic_group_psychotherapy Accessed: 17th August 2014.

Pilgrim, D., Rogers, A. and Bentall, R. (2009) 'The Centrality of Personal Relationships in the Creation and Amelioration of Mental Health Problems: The Current Interdisciplinary Case' *Health: An Interdisciplinary Journal for the Social Study of Health, Illness and Medicine* 13:2, 235–254.

Polanyi, M. (1966) *The Tacit Dimension*, Garden City, NY: Doubleday and Co.

Ricoeur, P. (1970) *Freud and Philosophy: An Essay on Interpretation* (trans. D. Savage) New Haven, CT: Yale University Press.

Rizq, R. (2013) 'IAPT and thought Crime: Language, Bureaucracy and the Evidence-based Regime' *Counselling Psychology Review*, 28:4, 111–115.

Snell. (2007) *L'Anti-Livre Noir de la Psychanalyse* Jacques-Alain Miller (ed) Reviewed in: *European Journal of Psychotherapy and Counselling*, June, 9:2, 231–239.

Verhaeghe, P. (2014) 'Neoliberalism has brought Out the Worst in Us' *The Guardian* 29th September 2014.

Vygotsky, L.S. (1962) *Thought and Language* Cambridge, MA: MIT Press.

Wittgenstein, L. (1958) *The Blue and Brown Books*, R. Rhees (ed) Oxford: Blackwell.

Index

Note: Page numbers followed by "n" denote endnotes.

Abraham, Karl 15
accountability 41–4, 49, 57
active imagination 16
Ajase, Prince 81–2
Akhtar, S. 123
Albee, G. W. 113
Alcohol, Drug Abuse and Mental Health Administration (ADAMHA) 52, 53
Alma Ata conference 113
Amaral, Tarsila do 70, 73n7
American psychoanalysis 107
American Psychological Association 43, 52
amnesia 67
Anderson, W. 110–11
Andrade, Mario de 68, 69, 73n6
Andrade, Oswald de 68–71, 73n4
anthropophagy 70–2
The Association for Psychohistory 95
Association of Child Psychotherapists (ACP) 142
Asylum Journal 8
asymmetry postulate 93–5
Augustine of Hippo 78, 106

barbarism 65, 66
Beck, Aaron T. 2, 19–20, 41, 58n12, 107; manual for CTOD 42–50 (see also cognitive therapy of depression (CTOD))
Being and Time (Heidegger) 19
Bekhterev, Vladimir 31
Berlin society 15
Berlin Wall 27, 34
Bernheim, Hippolyte 9, 11–13, 17
Beveridge, Craig 96
Bion, Wilfred 31, 137
black box (Latour) 42

Bleuler, Eugen 14–15
Bloor, David 93, 94
Borch-Jacobsen, M. 106
Bose, Jagadish Chandra 109, 122, 123, 127
Brady, John Paul 44
brain-storming 47
Brazil 5, 64, 66–9, 71, 110, 125
Brazilian alienism: anthropophagy 70–2; communism 71; critical consciousness 65; enlightenment thinking 64–5; liberation 71–2; Minas Gerais separatist conspiracy 68–9; Modern Art Week 68–9; modernity 66–7; primitivism 66
Brazilianness 68, 71
Brazil, Russia, India and China (BRIC) 125
Breuer, Josef 13
British Association for Counselling and Psychotherapy (BACP) 142
British Psychoanalytic Council (BPC) 142
Broad Spectrum Psychotherapy 44
Brokman, Aleksandra 33
Brown, Callum 97–9
Brown, Gordon 1
Buddhism 5, 78, 80–5, 87
Bykov, Konstantin 31

Calvinist Christianity 85
Camus, Jean 11
Carter, J. 41, 52
Catholic church 106
CBT see cognitive behaviour therapy (CBT)
Chakrabarty, Dipesh 3, 106, 126
Charcot, Jean-Martin 9, 12, 13
Chartier, R. 72
Chikazumi Jōkan 82–3
Children's House (Detski Dom) experiment 28

China 125, 127
Christianity 5, 78, 85, 87; apologetics 92;
    Brown's 97; Calvinist 85.; discursive
    92; Protestant 85; see also Scottish
    psychotherapy
Civilisation and its Discontents (Freud) 15
civilization 65
Clark, David M. 1, 2, 46
Clinical vs. Statistical Prediction
    (Meehl) 56
clinician and experiment 54–6
cognitive behaviour therapy (CBT) 1, 2,
    41, 107, 129, 130, 134–7, 141–5
cognitive therapy (CT) 20, 41, 44–6, 54,
    55, 107
Cognitive Therapy and the Emotional
    Disorders (Beck) 19
Cognitive Therapy Checklist 55
cognitive therapy of depression (CTOD)
    40–2, 57; clinician and experiment
    54–6; Klerman, Gerald 50–4; manual
    for 42–50; NIMH 50–4
Cohen, A. P. 96
Cold War 27, 34
collaboration 46
collectivism 30
colonialism 67
communism 27, 29, 35, 71
conditioned reflexes 31–2
'connected histories' 11
context of discovery 96
Craig, Carol 95–6
critical consciousness 65
Critical Psychotherapy, Psychoanalysis
    and Counselling: Implications for
    Practice (Loewenthal) 143, 145
CT see cognitive therapy (CT)
CTOD see cognitive therapy of
    depression (CTOD)
cultural practices 136–9
culture of manualisation 127–30
Czechoslovakia 28, 31, 33, 35

Davies, James 136
Delboeuf, Joseph 9–10, 20
democracy 42
Dendy, Walter Cooper 8
Deutsch, Helene 98
discursive bereavement 97, 98
discursive Christianity 92
Douste-Blazy, Philippe 138, 142
DSM-III diagnostic categories 53, 57
Dubois, Paul 10, 11, 33, 105, 108

Eastern Europe 108–9
East Germany 28, 30, 32
The Eclipse of Scottish Culture
    (Turnbull and Beveridge) 96
Egan, G. 129, 130
Ellenberger, H. F. 106
Ellis, Albert 34, 107
empirical investigation 49
enlightenment thinking 64–5
enthusiasm 108
European borderlands 107–8
European colonialism 67
European Enlightenment 126
The European Journal of Psychotherapy
    and Counselling 4
European model of civilization 72
Evidence-Based Medicine (EBM) 57
evidence-based research 138
existential psychotherapies 18
external reality 34

Facchinetti, Cristiana 5, 110, 122, 123
Fairbairn, W. R. D. 94
Falzeder, Ernst 14
Fanon, Frantz 96, 97
Ferenczi, Sandor 29
Food and Drug Administration (FDA) 41
Forel, August 14
Foucault, M. 106, 143
Foulkes, S. H. 31
Freud, Sigmund 13–16, 27, 65, 80, 82, 98,
    105, 106, 109–11, 121, 123, 127, 135
The Future of an Illusion (Freud) 15

Gauguin, Paul 66
General Resume of Techniques 45
Gergen, Kenneth 98
Gestalt therapy 19
Gjuričova, Adela 35
global psychotherapy 109–10, 123–6
gold standard research method 142
Goodman, Paul 19
grand hypnotisme 9
Granek, Leeat 98
Grof, Stanislav 29
Group of 5 71
Guideline Development Group
    (GDG) 140–1
guilt and religion 80

Harding, Christopher 109, 111, 122, 128
Hefferline, Ralph 19
Heidegger 19

Heisaku, Kosawa 109, 122, 128; buddhism and psychotherapy 80–5; religion-psy dialogue 85–8
Heller , A. 108
Hillman, J. 112
Hock, Kurt 30
Hoesterey, J. B. 111
Hollingshead , A. B. 113
'Homo Brasiliensis' 66–7
Horney, Karen 17
Huang , H.-Y. 111
hypnosis 10–11
hypnotic psycho-therapeutic 10

Illustrations of the Influence of the Mind Upon the Body in Health and Disease Designed to Elucidate the Action of the Imagination (Tuke) 8–9
implicit psychologies 97–9
Improving Access to Psychological Therapies (IAPT) 1, 2, 129, 130, 139, 141, 143, 144
Industrial Revolution 124
institutionalisation 15
Intentional Dynamic Group Psychotherapy 30
International Psycho-Analtyic Association 14, 28
International Society for Medical Psychology and Psychotherapy 14
Interpersonal Therapy (IPT) 51
Iron Curtain 27, 34

Janet, Pierre 12–13
Japanese Buddhism 85
Jaspers, Karl 8
Jena clinic 32
Jenson, D. 110–11
Jones, E. 105
The Journal of Psychohistory 95
Judeo-Christian religions 71
Jung, Carl Gustav 14–17, 29, 109

Kakar, S. 122
Keller , R. 110–11
Khatami, Manoocheer 44–6
Kierkegaard 19
Kleinman, Arthur 20
Klein, Melanie 80, 135
Kleinsorge, Helmuth 32
Klerman, Gerald 50–4
Klumbies, Gerhard 32
Kokorina, Marina 29–30

Kovacs, Maria 46–8
Kuhn, Thomas 50

Lacan, Jacques 107
Laing, R. D. 92, 97–9
Lasch, Christopher 78
Latour, Bruno 42
Layard, R. 144
Layard, Richard 1, 2, 6n2, 136
Lazarus, Arnold 44
Lears, Jackson 18
Lectures on Insanity (Winslow) 8
legitimacy 57n1
Lenin , V. I. 28, 29, 33, 34
Leuenberger, Christine 30
liberation 71–2
Liber Novus (Jung) 16
Liébault, Auguste Ambroise 9, 11
Linstrum, E. 110
Loewenthal, Del 5
Luborsky, Lester 44, 46, 53, 54
Luther, Martin 50

McLuhan, Marshall 20
Macunaima 68–9
Magalhaes, Couto de 73n10, 73n11
'Manifesto' 50, 67, 68, 70, 73n10, 73n11
manualisation of culture 127–30
Marks, Sarah 108, 130
Marxism 65, 71, 86
Marxist collectivism 31
Marxist–Leninist philosophers 27, 29
Maslow, A. H. 111
Materialism and Empirio - Criticism (Lenin) 34
Matza, T. 125
Mauss, M. 123
May, Rollo 18–19
Meehl, Paul 56
Mendels, Joe 45
mental health 1–3, 28, 52, 82, 106, 112–14, 136, 140, 142, 144
mental hygienists 113
mental illness 113
La mentalité primitive (1922) 73n8
The Mental States of Hysterics (Charcot) 12
Merleau-Ponty, M. 138
metanoia 92
Miassischev 30, 31, 33
middle class 124
Middleton, H. 140
Miller , M. A. 107, 108, 111, 131

Minas Gerais separatist conspiracy (1789) 68–9, 73n5
Minuchin, Salvador 44
mistaken approach 94
Modern Art Week (1922) 68–9
modernism 65, 66, 68, 71
modernity 66–7
Mood Clinic 46, 47
Moore, H. 122
moralism 92, 107
'Moral Treatment' 29
Moreira, Juliano 64, 72n1
Moreno, Jacob 31
Multimodal Therapy 44

Namu - Amida - Butsu: 'Hail to Amida Buddha' 83
National Institute for Health and Care Excellence (NICE) 5, 134–6, 138–42, 144
Neisser, Ulrich 97–8
Neurosis and Human Growth: The Struggle Toward Self Realization (Horney) 17
New Public Management 143
Nietzsche 65
NIMH administrators 50–4
North America 107

O'Donnell, J. M. 111
OECD 124
Orne, Martin 44
Ottawa charter for Health Promotion 113

Pagniez, Philippe 11
Parloff, Morris 51, 52, 54
passionate attitudes 13
Pau-Brasil Manifesto (1924) 67–9
Pavlov, Ivan 31, 32
Perls, Frederick 19
persuasion 33–4
Pessoa, Fernando 66, 72n2
Pfister, Oskar 111
Philadelphia 43–4
Platonov, Konstantin 32
Plotkin, Mariano Ben 110
Poland 33
Polanyi, M. 137
political character 30
political modernity 126
positive psychology 96
primitivism 66
private psychotherapy 124
Protestant Christianity 85

Protocol for Cognitive Behavioral Therapy of Depression: Rough draft 45
provincialisation 126–7
Provincializing Europe (Chakrabarty) 126
Psyche: A Discourse on the Birth and Pilgrimage of Thought (Dendy) 8
On the Psychical Mechanism of Hysteria: Preliminary Communication (Breuer) 13
psychoanalysis 15, 27–9, 84
psychoanalysts 110
psychoanalytic cosmologies 110–11
psychoanalytic discourse 98
psychoanalytic literature 14
'psycho-analytic purification' 15
psychoanalytic training system 15
psycho-diagnosis 66–7
psychodrama 31
psychohistory 95–6, 99
Psychological Automatism (Janet) 12
Psychological Medications (Janet) 13
psychological therapies, cultural practices 136–7
psychologies, implicit 97–9
psychologized assumptions 98
Psychoneuroses and Their Moral Treatment (Dubois) 10
psychopathology 16
The Psychopathology of Everyday Life (Freud) 15
psychotherapeia 8
psycho-therapeutic action 10
psychotherapeutic literature 14
psychotherapeutic procedure 15–16
psycho-therapeutics 8
Psycho-Therapeutics – Practical Applications of the Influence of the Mind on the Body to Medical Practice (Tuke) 9
psychotherapies 18, 20
psychotherapists 105, 111
psychotherapy: defined 2, 8; futility of 113; history of 11, 12; malleability of 18; scientific revolution 48

randomized-controlled trial (RCT) 41, 42, 45, 52–5, 57, 135–40, 142, 144
Rational Emotive Behaviour Therapy (REBT) 34, 130
Rational-Emotive Therapy 107
rational therapy 33–4, 107
reality principle 19
The Red Book (Jung) 16
Redlich , F. C. 113
Reich, Wilhelm 28

religion 111–12
religion-psy dialogue 85–8
religious 80
'Rest of the World' 106
Rickels, Karl 46
Ricoeur, P. 145
Rieff, Philip 78
Rizq, R. 146
Rogers, Carl 17–18, 31, 85, 86, 111, 127–9
Rose, Nikolas 77–8
Rosner, Rachel 19
Rudnick, L. 108
Rushforth, Winifred 92, 97, 99
Rush, John 44–50, 54, 58n12
Russia 29–30, 125

Sartre 19
The Savage (de Magalhaes) 73n10, 73n11
Savelli, Mat 31
Schmidt, Vera 28
Scotland 107–8
The Scots' Crisis of Confidence (Craig) 95
Scottish Protestantism 107, 108
Scottish psychotherapy 91–3,
    99–100; implicit psychologies
    97–9; and psychohistory 95–6;
    symmetrical vs. asymmetrical
    style 93–5
'Scrutinising NICE' (2012) 138, 139,
    141, 142
seduction theory 14
selflessness 79
self-realisation 17
Shamdasani, Sonu 146
Shaw, Brian 47, 48
Shellshock 17
Shin Buddhism 85, 109
Sirotkina, Irina 29–30
'small revolution in psychotherapy
    research' 54
socialism 29–32, 35
'socialist' psychotherapy 30
Society for Psychotherapy Research
    (SPR) 42
Soviet Union 27–35
The Structure of Scientific Revolutions
    (Kuhn) 50
Strupp, Hans 53, 54
subjectification 98
suggestive effect 10
supernaturalism 92, 107
Sutcliffe, Steven 97
Suzuki, Akihito 5

Suzuki, D. T. 85, 109
symmetry postulate 92, 93–5
Systems course 44
Szasz, Thomas 8

Taylor, E. 109
Tetsurō, Watsuji 86
'theory-lite' psychotherapies 17
theory of reflection (Lenin) 33
therapeutic ethos 18
Thrive: The Power of Evidence-Based
    Psychological Therapies (Clark and
    Layard) 1
Tillich, Paul 85–7, 111
Totem and Taboo (Freud) 111
'Tower of Babel' 14
The Transcendent Function (Jung) 16
trans-cultural dissemination 104–6,
    112–14; European borderlands
    107–8; global psychotherapy
    109–10; North America 107;
    psychoanalytic cosmologies 110–11;
    religion 111–12
transcultural histories 121, 130–1;
    culture of manualisation 127–30;
    global psychotherapy 123–6;
    manualisation of culture 127–30;
    provincialisation 126–7; universal
    truth 122–3
Treatment Assessment Research
    (TAR) 52
Treatment Manual for Cognitive-
    Behavioral Therapy of Depression 45
Treatment of Depression Collaborative
    Research Program (TDCRP) 52–4
Trump, Donald 95
Tuke, Daniel Hack 8–10
Tummala-Narra, P. 123
Turnbull, Ronald 96

United Kingdom (UK) 134
United Kingdom Council for
    Psychotherapy (UKCP) 138
universal truth 122–3
Utopia 72

Vaihinger, Hans 94
van Eeden, Frederick 8
Ventura, M. 112
Verhaeghe, P. 144
Vivekananda, Swami 109
Vos, Jan de 78
Vygotsky, L. S. 138

Waskow, Irene 51, 52, 54
Weber 71
Weissman, Myrna 50, 51
Western discipline 121
Western theory and practice 125–6
Winnicott, Donald 80
Winslow, Forbes 8
Wisdom, Madness and Folly (Laing) 97
Wittgenstein, L. 136
Wolpe, Joseph 44
*The Word as a Physiological
   and Therapeutic Factor:*

*The Theory and Practice of
Psychotherapy According to
I.P. Pavlov* (Platonov) 32
work therapy 29–30
World Health Organisation 113
Wright, R. 111

Yogananda, Paramahansa 109
Yogi, Maharishi Mahesh 109
Yugoslavia 29

Zhang, L. 125

For Product Safety Concerns and Information please contact our EU
representative GPSR@taylorandfrancis.com
Taylor & Francis Verlag GmbH, Kaufingerstraße 24, 80331 München, Germany